Skin Cancer

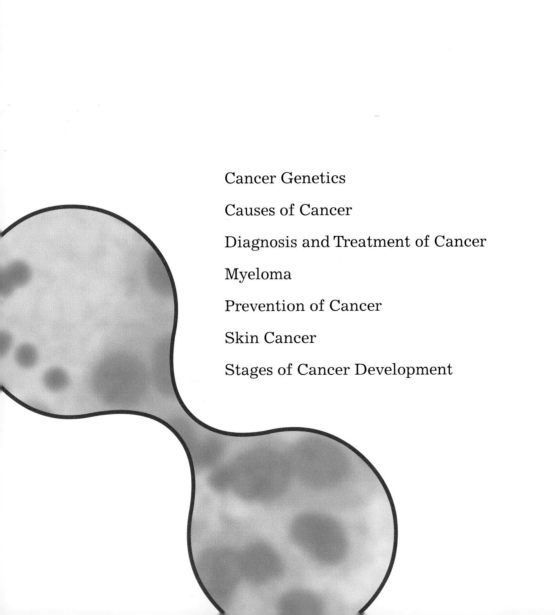

Skin Cancer

Po-Lin So, Ph.D.

Consulting Editor,
Donna M. Bozzone, Ph.D.
Professor of Biology
Saint Michael's College

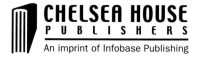

CHELSEA HOUSE
PUBLISHERS
An imprint of Infobase Publishing

THE BIOLOGY OF CANCER: SKIN CANCER

Chelsea House
An imprint of Infobase Publishing
132 West 31st Street
New York NY 10001

Library of Congress Cataloging-in-Publication Data
So, Po-Lin.
  Skin cancer / Po-Lin So.
     p. cm. – (Biology of cancer)
  Includes bibliographical references and index.
  ISBN-13: 978-0-7910-8938-5
  ISBN-10: 0-7910-8938-X
  1. Skin–Cancer–Popular works. I. Title. II. Series.

  RC280.S5S6 2008
  616.99'477–dc22

                                        2007027470

Chelsea House books are available at special discounts when purchased in bulk quantities for businesses, associations, institutions, or sales promotions. Please call our Special Sales Department in New York at (212) 967-8800 or (800) 322-8755.

You can find Chelsea House on the World Wide Web at http://www.chelseahouse.com

Text design by James Scotto-Lavino
Cover design by Ben Peterson

Printed in the United States of America

Bang EJB 10 9 8 7 6 5 4 3 2 1

This book is printed on acid-free paper.

All links and Web addresses were checked and verified to be correct at the time of publication. Because of the dynamic nature of the Web, some addresses and links may have changed since publication and may no longer be valid.

Avastin® is a registered trademark of Genentech, Inc. Tazorac® is a registered trademark of Allergan, Inc.

CONTENTS

◆

FOREWORD

◆

Approximately 1,500 people die each day of cancer in the United States. Worldwide, more than 8 million new cases are diagnosed each year. In affluent, developed nations such as the United States, around one out of three people will develop cancer in his or her lifetime. As deaths from infection and malnutrition become less prevalent in developing areas of the world, people live longer and cancer incidence increases to become a leading cause of mortality. Clearly, few people are left untouched by this disease due either to their own illness or that of loved ones. This situation leaves us with many questions: What causes cancer? Can we prevent it? Is there a cure?

Cancer did not originate in the modern world. Evidence of humans afflicted with cancer dates from ancient times. Examinations of bones from skeletons that are more than 3,000 years old reveal structures that appear to be tumors. Records from ancient Egypt, written more than 4,000 years ago, describe breast cancers. Possible cases of bone tumors have been observed in Egyptian mummies that are more than 5,000 years old. It is even possible that our species' ancestors developed cancer. In 1932, Louis Leakey discovered a jawbone, from either *Australopithecus* or *Homo erectus*, that possessed what appeared to be a tumor. Cancer specialists examined the jawbone and suggested that the tumor was due to Burkitt's lymphoma, a type of cancer that affects the immune system.

It is likely that cancer has been a concern for the human lineage for at least a million years.

Human beings have been searching for ways to treat and cure cancer since ancient times, but cancer is becoming an even greater problem today. Because life expectancy increased dramatically in the twentieth century due to public health successes such as improvements in our ability to prevent and fight infectious disease, more people live long enough to develop cancer. Children and young adults can develop cancer, but the chance of developing the disease increases as a person ages. Now that so many people live longer, cancer incidence has increased dramatically in the population. As a consequence, the prevalence of cancer came to the forefront as a public health concern by the middle of the twentieth century. In 1971 President Richard Nixon signed the National Cancer Act and thus declared "war" on cancer. The National Cancer Act brought cancer research to the forefront and provided funding and a mandate to spur research to the National Cancer Institute. During the years since that action, research laboratories have made significant progress toward understanding cancer. Surprisingly, the most dramatic insights came from learning how normal cells function, and by comparing that to what goes wrong in cancer cells.

Many people think of cancer as a single disease, but it actually comprises more than 100 different disorders in normal cell and tissue function. Nevertheless, all cancers have one feature in common: All are diseases of uncontrolled cell division. Under normal circumstances, the body regulates the production of new cells very precisely. In cancer cells, particular defects in deoxyribonucleic acid, or DNA, lead to breakdowns in the cell communication and growth control that are normal in healthy cells. Having escaped these controls, cancer cells can become invasive and spread to other parts of the body. As a consequence, normal tissue and organ functions may be seriously disrupted. Ultimately, cancer can be fatal.

Even though cancer is a serious disease, modern research has provided many reasons to feel hopeful about the future of cancer treatment and prevention. First, scientists have learned a great deal about the specific genes involved in cancer. This information paves the way for improved early detection, such as identifying individuals with a genetic predisposition to cancer and monitoring their health to ensure the earliest possible detection. Second, knowledge of both the specific genes involved in cancer and the proteins made by cancer cells has made it possible to develop very specific and effective treatments for certain cancers. For example, childhood leukemia, once almost certainly fatal, now can be treated successfully in the great majority of cases. Similarly, improved understanding of cancer cell proteins led to the development of new anticancer drugs such as Herceptin, which is used to treat certain types of breast tumors. Third, many cancers are preventable. In fact, it is likely that more than 50 percent of cancers would never occur if people avoided smoking, overexposure to sun, a high-fat diet, and a sedentary lifestyle. People have tremendous power to reduce their chances of developing cancer by making good health and lifestyle decisions. Even if treatments become perfect, prevention is still preferable to avoid the anxiety of a diagnosis and the potential pain of treatment.

The books in *The Biology of Cancer* series reveal information about the causes of the disease; the DNA changes that result in tumor formation; ways to prevent, detect, and treat cancer; and detailed accounts of specific types of cancers that occur in particular tissues or organs. Books in this series describe what happens to cells as they lose growth control and how specific cancers affect the body. *The Biology of Cancer* series also provides insights into the studies undertaken, the research experiments done, and the scientists involved in the development of the present state of knowledge of this disease. In this way, readers get to see beyond "the facts" and understand more about the process of biomedical research. Finally, the books in *The Biology of Cancer* series provide information to help readers make healthy choices that can reduce the risk of cancer.

Cancer research is at a very exciting crossroads, affording scientists the challenge of scientific problem solving as well as the opportunity to engage in work that is likely to directly benefit people's health and well-being. I hope that the books in this series will help readers learn about cancer. Even more, I hope that these books will capture your interest and awaken your curiosity about cancer so that you ask questions for which scientists presently have no answers. Perhaps some of your questions will inspire you to follow your own path of discovery. If so, I look forward to your joining the community of scientists; after all, there is still a lot of work to be done.

Donna M. Bozzone, Ph.D.
Professor of Biology
Saint Michael's College
Colchester, Vermont

1

INTRODUCTION TO CANCER

KEY POINTS

- Cancer is the second biggest killer in the United States. Anyone can develop cancer, and the older we are, the more likely we are to develop the disease.

- Cancer is a multistep process that begins when genetic mutations in normal cells cause them to grow uncontrollably.

- Our genes are a major factor that determine whether we will develop cancer, but environmental factors can increase our chances of developing cancer.

- Cancer is a collection of diseases and one cancer may behave very differently from another. Cancers can be nonlife-threatening (benign) or life-threatening (malignant).

- Early-stage cancers are easier to treat than late-stage cancers. Cancer that has spread to other parts of the body is generally difficult, if not impossible, to treat.

Almost everyone has heard of someone who has had cancer. The word itself strikes fear in our hearts since we know that this group of diseases can be highly aggressive and in the worst-case scenario, cancer can kill a person relatively quickly, often in a painful way. In 2006, Dana Reeve, the American actress and wife of the late Christopher Reeve (famous for his "Superman" movies and for his pioneering spirit after he broke his neck falling from a horse), died of lung cancer at age 44, within a year of her **diagnosis**. She had been responding well to treatment and was looking fairly healthy only a couple of months before she succumbed to her cancer. Another celebrity who also recently died of lung cancer was the American-Canadian journalist and anchorman for ABC News, Peter Jennings. His lung cancer was probably caused by his lifetime of smoking. He died about four months after his diagnosis.

Despite these tragic cases, not everyone dies soon after developing cancer. A remarkable story of cancer survival is the one of Lance Armstrong, the world-renowned American cyclist who won the prestigious Tour de France an unprecedented seven straight times, from 1999 to 2005, a couple of years after he was diagnosed with testicular cancer (cancer of the testicles). In his book, *It's Not About the Bike: My Journey Back to Life*, he describes his experience with the disease and even goes as far to suggest that the cancer treatment he endured dramatically "remodeled" his physique (by reducing his body mass), which helped his cycling performance over the mountains of the Pyrenees and the Alps!

Armstrong's spectacular sporting achievements are unique to him; however, getting cancer is not. Not everyone is as lucky to survive and live a relatively "normal" life, or even an extraordinary life like Armstrong's. Indeed, cancer is the second leading cause of death in the United States (heart disease is the number one killer). It afflicts all ages, from young to old. Cancer, however, is mainly a disease of older people since it generally takes many years for it to develop. So the longer we live, the more likely we are to develop cancer. Nearly half of all men and a little over one-third of all women in the United States will develop cancer at some point during their lifetime. At present, there are few cures for those cancers that have spread throughout the body (metastasized); however, if the cancer is detected early and treated immediately, there is a better chance of surviving the disease.

CANCER TERMINOLOGY

Cancer as a disease has been documented as far back as 1600 B.C. by the ancient Egyptians. It was the Greek physician Hippocrates, however, in 400 B.C., who used the Greek word *karkinoma*, meaning crab, to describe the way the long projections of cancer cells "claw" their way down into the tissue and organs, like crabs clawing their way down a sandy beach. The Roman author and encyclopedia writer Aulus Cornelius Celsus (25 B.C.) translated this Greek term for crab into its Latin version—*cancer*—which is the common term we use today. A word similar to *karkinoma*, **carcinoma**, is often used to describe cancers that develop from the outer lining of tissues and organs, the **epithelium**, such as basal cell carcinoma (a skin cancer) and renal cell carcinoma (a kidney cancer). Most cancers form solid masses, or **tumors**, at their primary location. The word tumor comes from Latin and means "swelling." Not all cancers start as solid tumor masses: Cancers of the blood, such as leukemia, do not form primary tumors. Instead, they circulate through the cardiovascular and **lymphatic systems** to other tissues; if they "take root" there, the cancer will then grow as solid secondary tumors, also known as **metastases**. The term, **carcinogen**, which is

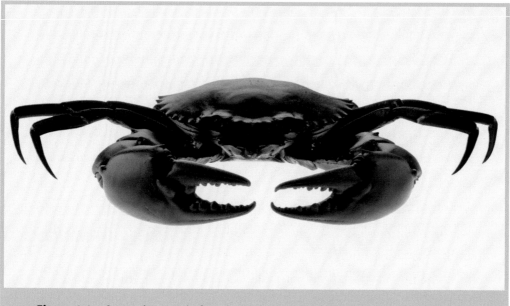

Figure 1.1   Cancer is named after the crab. *(Mohd Fadhil Kamarundin/iStockphoto)*

related to carcinoma, is used to describe environmental agents that may increase a person's chances of developing cancer.

Professionals who study and/or treat cancer may use other terms, such **malignancy** and **neoplasm**, to describe a cancerous growth. The field of cancer is generally referred to as **oncology**, which is derived from the Greek word for mass (or tumor)—*onkos*—and the suffix *ology*, which means "study of." An **oncologist** is a professional who specializes in treating cancer.

WHAT IS CANCER?

Cancer is often thought of as one disease, but it is actually a collection of diseases that develops from normal cells through a multistep process.

Different types of cancer generally behave very differently. For example, they may be caused by different **genetic mutations** (changes from the normal **genetic code**), grow at different rates, and/or respond to different treatments. This is even true for cancers that develop from the same type of cell in the same organ. Therefore, cancer is a highly complex group of diseases and it is important to understand as much as possible about each type of cancer to be able to treat this group of dreadful diseases effectively.

From the start of a person's life, cells grow and divide (proliferate) rapidly until adulthood, when cell proliferation becomes restricted to only the parts of the body that require constant cellular renewal (such as the skin, intestine, and hair follicles, for example). The need for cellular renewal is because our bodies undergo general "wear and tear" all the time, and often we get an injury (for example, from falling over) that requires damaged and dying cells to be replaced constantly to keep the organs healthy and functional. Cellular renewal in the body needs to be strictly regulated to ensure that enough cells are made to replace the old, damaged, or dying cells, but also to make sure that not too many cells are made, since that would be inefficient and energy-consuming. All cells have a built-in sensor system that detects cellular and genetic damage. When damage is detected, the cell will try to repair itself. If the damage is too great to be repaired, however, the cell instructs itself to stop growing and to initiate its built-in "self-destruct" program. This process is called programmed cell death, or **apoptosis**.

Cancer is caused by abnormal, "out-of-control" cells that have acquired the ability to sneak past all the checkpoints for growth control and apoptosis to essentially become immortal. These abnormal cells proliferate uncontrollably and change their form to become even more aggressive, abnormal cells that are genetically unstable (i.e., the genetic information is even more damaged) and, accumulate more **deleterious** (damaging) genetic mutations. Some of these **mutations** may give some of the cancer cells the ability to escape and spread to other parts of the body through the lymphatic system and/or the bloodstream. Once they have spread, they may take root in other organs and start growing rapidly, damaging the host organ's cells and disrupting their normal function. If the cancer spreads throughout the body, it becomes a life-threatening cancer. The process in which cancer cells break away from the original cancer mass and establish new tumor sites in other organs is called **metastasis**. If metastasis of a cancer has occurred in a patient, it is generally very difficult, if not impossible, to cure.

Although cancer is a worldwide disease that affects many people, overall it is remarkably rare given that there are many cells proliferating in our bodies at any given time. The sheer number of cells in our bodies (between 50 trillion and 100 trillion—that's 50 million million to 100 million million cells!) provides numerous chances for mistakes to happen in the underlying cell processes. Yet the transformation of healthy cells into cancerous cells is a rare event. Therefore, what is surprising is not that cancer afflicts so many people, but that it strikes so few.

THE HALLMARKS OF CANCER

In 2000, two renowned U.S. cancer biologists, Douglas Hanahan (at the University of California, San Francisco) and Robert Weinberg (at the Whitehead Institute for Biomedical Research, Massachusetts Institute of Technology) outlined in a scientific paper, the six specific characteristics that most cancers possess. In general, cancers:

1. Have the ability to grow indefinitely—they have limitless replicative potential.

2. Are able to ignore the anti-cell-growth signals that tell cells to stop dividing.

3. Are able to evade the signals that tell them to undergo apoptosis (self-destruction).

4. Have the ability to make "self-sustaining" factors to promote their own growth.

5. Are able to recruit other cells to make a network of new blood vessels to sustain themselves—this process is known as **angiogenesis**.

6. Can invade other tissues and cause new tumor growth.

WHO GETS CANCER?

Anyone can develop cancer, since we all have cells that are constantly undergoing cellular processes such as proliferation and apoptosis to replace old, damaged, and dying cells, and DNA to repair or "fix" genetic information that have been damaged by environmental factors. If there is a malfunction in any of these processes, cancer can occur. Some people are more likely to develop cancer than others because their genetic makeup makes them more susceptible. Indeed, we have all heard the stories of cigarette smokers who died of lung cancer in their 50s countered with the stories of granddad, who smoked all his life and died from natural causes at age 90.

At the most basic level, cancer is a "disease of **genes**." Genes are units of genetic information. Some gene mutations can directly cause cancer and are deleterious mutations. Other gene mutations, such as genetic **polymorphisms** may increase the chances of some of us getting cancer if we are exposed to a carcinogen. As mentioned above, a common carcinogen is cigarette smoke, which can significantly increase our chance of developing lung cancer if we smoke throughout our lifetime.

GENETICS OF CANCER SUSCEPTIBILITY

Inherited Cancer

Cancer can develop from a germline mutation. This is when the person inherits a damaged (or mutant) copy of a gene from his or her parents and has a much higher probability of developing the disease than a person who does not have the inherited gene mutation. Inherited mutations that substantially increase a person's risk of getting cancer include mutations in *BRCA1*, which can cause breast cancer, and *PATCHED1*, which results in many basal cell carcinomas in these people. These direct, cancer-causing, **familial** mutations are generally unusual, develop relatively early compared to sporadic cancers, and account for no more than 2 to 5 percent of all cancers. All other cancers are noninherited, sporadic cancers (below) and are caused by gene mutations that arise spontaneously in a person's lifetime.

The deleterious gene mutation will code for a protein that may have abnormal function or no function. In these situations the cell can no longer function normally. Gene mutations may be dominant or recessive. That is, if a person inherits one copy of the mutated gene and it is dominant, he or she will develop the disease. On the other hand, if the gene mutation is recessive, the person will only develop the disease if he or she inherits two copies of the mutation.

Sporadic Cancer

Cancers that arise spontaneously (i.e., not because of an inherited genetic mutation but because of a spontaneous genetic mutations in

---

◆ AUTOSOMAL AND SEX-LINKED CHROMOSOMAL INHERITANCE

All people have 46 **chromosomes** in every cell of their bodies except for sperm and egg cells, which have 23 chromosomes, and mature red blood cells, which expel their nuclei (and therefore have no DNA) when they mature so that they are more efficient at carrying oxygen around the body. Chromosomes contain genes, which are distinct units of DNA that contains the information to make specific proteins. Each of us has 22 pairs of nonsex, or **autosomal**, chromosomes and one pair of sex chromosomes, which determine whether someone is male or female: Females have two X chromosomes and males have one X and one Y chromosome. Autosomal diseases, such as basal cell carcinoma and cystic fibrosis (a disease of the lungs), are inherited through the nonsex chromosomes, while sex-linked diseases, such as color blindness and hemophilia (a blood-clotting disorder) are inherited through the sex chromosomes.

---

a person's lifetime) are called "sporadic cancers." Sporadic cancers mainly develop from epithelial cells, the cells that line tissues or vessels. Epithelium can be found lining the internal organs (for example, the endothelium lines the inside of blood vessels) or external free surfaces (such as the epidermis, which is the outermost layer of the skin) of the body. More than 90 percent of cancers are epithelial cancers, which include **nonmelanoma skin cancer,** and are relatively common, since the epithelial layers of the skin are constantly undergoing repair and/or renewal. Other epithelial cancers include intestinal cancer, breast cancer and ovarian cancer.

In any population, there are a significant number of seemingly harmless genetic variations. These are neither good nor bad mutations and are part of normal genetic evolution, giving rise to the differences between individuals. However, some of these polymorphisms are coupled with a disease-causing gene mutation, they may influence the severity of the disease. If they are not coupled to a gene mutation, these variations can make us more susceptible to developing a disease that is determined largely by environmental factors.

The Influence of Behavior and Environment on Cancer

As already mentioned, most people do not have gene mutations that directly cause cancer, but have certain combinations of genetic polymorphisms that may increase their chances of getting cancer if exposed to environmental factors such as tobacco, alcohol, radiation, work-related toxins, infections, bad diet, and certain drugs. Of cancers that affect the colon, lung, breast, stomach, prostate, and skin, at least 65 percent can be traced to environmental carcinogens. These can be chemicals—for example, asbestos, which is used in building materials, causes a type of lung cancer called **mesothelioma**—or high energy radiation—for example, ultraviolet light and X rays cause skin cancer. A list of known and suspected carcinogens can be found on the Web site for the American Cancer Society (http://www.cancer.org). Environmental carcinogens damage cells and their DNA, which leads to gene mutations that cause cancer.

Where we live may also contribute significantly. For breast cancer, there is **epidemiological** data indicating that women born in Asia who immigrate to the United States as adults tend to develop breast cancer at about the same rate as their female counterparts back in Asia. Their granddaughters born in the United States, however, have breast cancer rates about 80 percent higher than their grandmothers who came from Asia (i.e., at levels similar to American-born women of European background). This increase of breast cancer in the Western world has been suggested to be due to differences in diet: In Japan, people eat less fatty foods and red meat, and more fish than people in the West. However, no one knows for sure how much influence a certain diet has on causing cancer.

Lifestyle choices can also determine whether a person might develop cancer. For example, most cases of lung cancer, which is the leading cause of cancer deaths in both men and women, can be attributed to smoking. Indeed, long-term smoking is most likely the cause of Peter Jennings' lung cancer. Therefore, to reduce the chances of developing smoking-related lung cancer, a person should not smoke and should avoid smoke-filled places.

Oncogenes and Tumor Suppressor Genes

Of the 30,000 genes in the human genome that code for different proteins, a few hundred genes regulate growth and are most active during the development of the embryo. Some of these "growth" genes promote cancer development and are called **oncogenes**. In cancer, mutations in oncogenes produce proteins that function in a way that is somewhat like a constantly depressed accelerator in a car, allowing cancer to grow out-of-control. An example of an oncogene is *Ras*, which is mutated in cancers of the pancreas, colon, and skin, resulting in its protein product being abnormally activated, causing the uncontrolled growth of cells that have the mutated protein.

Genes that prevent cancer development are called **tumor suppressor genes**. They normally produce proteins that act like car brakes, inhibiting the cell cycle and the birth of new cells and sometimes promoting apoptosis. If these "brake genes" are damaged, cancer can develop. Examples of a tumor suppressor gene is *p53*, which is arguably the most important tumor suppressor gene in cancer, and *PATCHED1*, which is mutated in basal cell nevus syndrome.

Gene Nomenclature

In biology, the names for human genes and proteins are generally written in capital letters, while the names of genes and protein for mice are generally in lowercase letters. All gene names are italicized and are given short symbols. The proteins that the genes code for are not italicized. For example, take the gene *Patched1*: the human gene

---

◆ THE *p53* TUMOR SUPPRESSOR GENE: "THE GUARDIAN OF THE GENOME"

The *p53* gene was the first tumor suppressor gene to be identified, in 1984. At first, it was thought to be an oncogene since experiments in which a *p53* gene sequence was introduced into cells immortalized with an "oncogenic *Ras*" gene proliferated much more than the same cells without the *p53* gene sequence. However, 10 years of extensive research showed that *p53* is in fact a tumor suppressor gene. The reason why greater cell proliferation was observed in those initial experiments was because the researchers unknowingly used a *p53* gene sequence that contained a mutation that changed its function.

P53 is so-called because the protein product "weighed" about 53 kilodaltons (a dalton is a unit of mass named after the British teacher and scientist John Dalton, who developed the first modern atomic theory in

and protein is *PATCHED1* (symbol: *PTCH1*) and PATCHED1 (symbol: PTCH1), respectively. The mouse gene and protein are *Patched1* (symbol: *Ptch1*) and Patched (symbol: Ptch1), respectively.

STAGES OF CANCER DEVELOPMENT

Cancer begins when a cell acquires damage to its **DNA (deoxyribonucleic acid)**. DNA is a double-stranded, helical chain of biological molecules that is found within the nucleus of each cell (except mature blood cells). It carries our genetic blueprint in the form of specific combinations of biological molecules called nucleotides, of which

1803). The normal function for p53 protein is DNA repair, cell-cycle arrest, and/or apoptosis. It functions by controlling a cell's entry into the cell division cycle. When a cell's DNA is damaged, the *p53* gene is induced and produces p53 protein that activates target genes that are involved in DNA repair. If the DNA is too damaged, p53 signals for the cell to commit suicide. Therefore, p53 protein is an important cell cycle regulator. In most cancers, p53 protein does not function correctly due to gene mutations. At least 50 percent of all these tumors have nonfunctional p53 protein due to mutations in the *p53* gene itself. In many other cancers, p53 is inactivated indirectly by viruses that use their viral proteins to bind to and block proteins that "stabilize" the p53 protein, causing it to lose its function. Also, mutations occur in genes that code for proteins that normally interact in the pathway that p53 protein functions. This may also result in the development of cancer. Therefore, many scientists believe that *p53* is the most important tumor suppressor gene.

there are four: adenine (A), thymidine (T), cytosine (C) and guanidine (G). This genetic blueprint carries all the information that makes us what we are. Genes are discrete units of DNA that code for proteins, the functional components of the cell that enable cells to reproduce and perform their functions.

DNA damage can be caused by a number of factors, including exposure to radiation, such as X rays and sunlight. In addition, **free radicals** (highly reactive chemicals that often contain oxygen) that are normally produced by the cell during normal biological processes can cause DNA damage if not cleared sufficiently within the cell. DNA damage is bad since it results in regions of DNA begin altered, which changes the genetic code. Deleterious gene mutations can cause cancer and other diseases since altered genes produce faulty proteins that do not function properly. Cancer is commonly initiated by mutations that affect genes that encode proteins, which regulate the cell cycle. Disruption of crucial cell cycle regulators can start a chain reaction of events that leads to cancer development.

Precancerous Cells "Go Wild"

The renegade "precancer" cell that has escaped death begins to proliferate out of control to form a clonal (identical) population of abnormal cells. This process is called **hyperplasia**. Some of these "hyperplastic" cells become even more genetically unstable, which leads to more genetic and cellular instability in the cells, making them even more abnormal (**dysplastic**). These dysplastic cells may then develop the ability to recruit surrounding normal cells and convert them to become part of what is now developing into a cancer. Some of these converted cells now form a specialized "extracellular matrix," or stroma, which acts as a structural framework for the cancer cells to develop in. It also provides the cancer cells with growth and survival signals to keep the cancer growing and to protect it from being attacked by the body's immune system, which may recognize the tumor as foreign. When cancer has developed to this level of organization, it has become a **primary tumor**.

When Cancer Takes Hold

The primary tumor is a well-defined structure made up of the initial cancerous cells and stromal cells, which help to support tumor growth. To further nourish itself, the tumor recruits surrounding cells to make a system of blood vessels (angiogenesis) that allows the blood to carry oxygen and other nutrients to feed the tumor. At this stage, the tumor is called a cancer *in situ* ("in the original position"—the cancer just sits in the site where it has developed). At this stage, it can follow one of two routes:

1. The Benign Route. The tumor may continue to grow uncontrollably as a **benign** (noncancerous) tumor. These tumors are generally not life-threatening. Benign tumors are usually removed by surgery to prevent a) the destruction of local cells; b) further complications, such as physical pressure on surrounding organs as the tumor grows; c) excess secretion of substances that the cancer cells may produce, which might interfere with the body's normal function—an example of a "secreting cancer" is adrenal adenoma, a benign glandular tumor of the adrenal gland that secretes high levels of the hormone aldosterone, causing headaches, weakness, fatigue, high blood salt levels, frequent urination, high blood pressure, and irregular heartbeats in the patient; and d) to prevent any chance of the benign tumor becoming a more aggressive cancer.

2. The Metastatic Route. The tumor may acquire even more damaging genetic mutations and develop into an aggressive (destructive) tumor,

which grows out-of-control, destroying the surrounding cells and tissues for its own selfish needs. During this process, the cells may undergo changes to acquire characteristics of another cell type. For example, an epithelial cancer cell may change into a more mesenchymal (a connective tissue-like) cancer cell type, which may give it the ability to escape to other regions of the body more easily. This process is called **metaplasia**. At this stage, the tumor and its stroma secrete proteins that can dissolve and break through the thin physical barrier that normally separates two different tissue layers—the **basement membrane**, allowing the tumor to spread and invade the surrounding tissues. This is known as invasive cancer and the tumor is on its way to becoming **malignant**. Invasive cancers shed hundreds to thousands of malignant cells, which travel via the blood and lymphatic system to other organs of the body, where they may grow uncontrollably and disrupt normal bodily functions. This metastasis is the event that causes most deaths from cancer. Although these metastases are found in other organs, they maintain many of the characteristics of the primary tumor from which they originated. It is important to realize this when treating a metastatic tumor, since some therapies are tumor-specific: In other words, they target the initial cancer cell type.

Metastasis

Metastasis is a word that people dread to hear. It indicates the worst kind of news when being diagnosed with cancer since it means that the cancer has spread around the body and, in most cases, will be very resistant to any kind of therapy. In many cases, metastasis will result in a rapid and painful death. Even after a successful treatment of a primary metastasis, the cancer may recur many years later to develop into an even more aggressive cancer that is nonresponsive to any treatments.

From Primary Cancer to Metastatic Cancer

For a cancer to become metastatic, it must undergo a series of steps. First, as a primary tumor, it needs to develop a blood supply to provide it with nutrients. This process of generating new blood vessels—angiogenesis—also provides an escape route for tumor cells that have "shed" from the primary growth site to enter the body's blood system. This process is known as intravasation. Another escape route is via the lymphatic system, which drains into the blood system. Once in circulation, the tumor cells need to survive. Survival occurs when the cancer cells acquire mutations that give them the power to fight off any would-be cellular attackers that may recognize the cancer cells as alien and want to destroy them. These defenders include components of the body's immune system. Alternatively, the cancer cells may fool the body's defense system into thinking they are harmless and the body's protectors leave them alone.

Once they reach a host organ, the tumor cells can either be rejected or accepted by their host. If the host organ is receptive to them, they may start to grow into secondary tumors, or **preangiogenic micrometastases**. It is thought that specific biological factors that are normally produced by the host organ can attract the circulating tumor cells. Different types of cancer have preferences for certain target organs. For example, breast cancer tends to metastasize to the **lymph nodes** under the arms, the brain, the bones, and the liver. Thus, tumor cells first escape via the lymphatic system and/or blood system and then home in on the organs that secrete the attractant molecules. Once the micrometastases

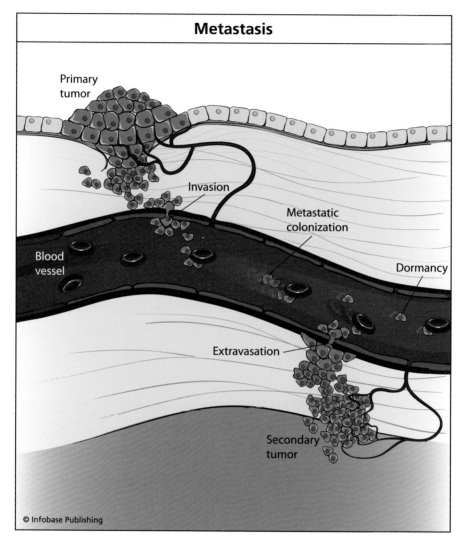

Metastasis

Primary tumor

Invasion

Metastatic colonization

Dormancy

Blood vessel

Extravasation

Secondary tumor

© Infobase Publishing

Figure 1.2   Metastasis requires shedding of primary tumor cells into the lymphatic and blood systems to secondary sites. After this movement of tumor cells to the distant site (extravasation), cells will either lie dormant (or "sleep"), die, or proliferate into a secondary cancer.

are developing in the attracting organ, angiogenesis is required to feed the tumor for it to develop into a **macroscopic** tumor (a tumor that is visible to the naked eye).

Detection of Metastases

Usually a person will go to see their doctor if they develop a lump on their body (for example, on the skin or in the breast) or if there is some medical problem such as unexplained loss of weight, or abnormal bowel stools, which can indicate colon cancer. The doctor may then carry out a series of tests, such as physical whole body examinations, cellular and biochemical tests (such as blood tests) and X ray scans, to see whether the patient has cancer. If cancer is suspected, the doctor may order a batch of tests to see whether the cancer has spread. The first point of call is the nearby lymph nodes. A sentinel lymph node (the lymph node closest to the primary tumor) **biopsy** is a standard procedure done to see whether a cancer has spread. A radioactive substance and blue dye are injected into the primary tumor region and the sentinel lymph node is checked for radioactivity an hour later. If no radioactivity is found, the cancer has not metastasized. If the node is radioactive and blue, however, it is removed and checked for metastases histologically (i.e., by examining the cellular organization). If cancer cells are found, the other lymph nodes in the area (the regional lymph nodes) are removed. Surgical (excisional) lymph node biopsy is another common method for checking whether the cancer has spread to nearby tissues lymph nodes. It is done if a lymph node is enlarged and involves removing the lymph node through a small incision. If the cancer is thought to have spread to other parts of the body, fine needle aspiration biopsy (FNA) is carried out. It involves the insertion of a small needle into a suspected metastatic region, such as an enlarged sentinel lymph node for example, to remove some of the cellular material. The technique is similar to drawing blood. The cells are then analyzed by oncologists and pathologists (doctors who identify diseases by studying cells and tissues under a microscope).

If metastasis to other organs is suspected, imaging procedures are also carried out. These procedures include chest X rays and computed tomography (CT) scans, which are done to see if the cancer has spread to the lungs and liver—common sites of advanced metastasis (when the cancer had spread all over the body). Many images are taken by the scanner and compiled by a computer to give detailed, cross-sectional views of the body. CT scans take longer than regular X rays since they require the patient to lie still for 15 to 30 minutes, but they give images of better resolution than an X ray. Another now-common way of imaging internal cancers is magnetic resonance imaging (MRI), which is like a CT scan except that it uses radio waves and strong magnets to produce an image. MRI scans are used especially for looking at soft tissue such as the brain and spinal cord. Another imaging techniques commonly used is positron emission tomography (PET). This technique uses a "radioactive sugar" to generate an image. These radioactive sugars are injected into the patient's vein and collect in regions of the body that have cancer since actively growing cancers have a high metabolic rate (they expend a lot of energy) and use up more sugars than normal tissues do. These high "radioactive sugar" regions can be spotted with the PET scanner. This technique is especially useful for finding internal metastatic tumors since they grow very fast and "light up" readily on PET scan.

Several cancers metastasize to the bone, so nuclear bone scans are used to detect these metastases. This is done by injecting small amounts of radioactive chemical tracers into a vein, which collects in the bone regions where the cancer has spread. This technique is not exclusive to cancer and is often used for detecting other conditions, such as arthritis, bone infections, and fractures.

Cancer Staging

Once cancer is detected, it is important for oncologists to "stage" the cancer. Knowing the stage will give the doctors a better idea of what treatment to give. This is essential if the cancer has metastatic potential. Cancer staging is based on a) the location of the primary tumor; b) the size and number of the tumors; c) the spread to lymph nodes; d) the cell type and how similar the cancer cells are to the normal tissue; and e) whether metastasis has occurred. A low stage number (for example, Stage I), indicates a less aggressive, more treatable cancer, while a higher stage (for example, Stage IV) indicates a cancer that is more aggressive, more out-of-control, and harder to treat. In general, less aggressive cancers resemble the more developed (i.e. differentiated) cells from the organ from which they arose, while more aggressive cancers are in the more "primitive" form—that is, they resemble less developed cell types of the organ from which they arose. The clinical staging systems may vary depending on the type of cancer. A general outline for staging cancer is as follows:

Stage 0 cancer is when the cancer is in its early development and is only present in the cell layer from which it developed. Stage I cancer is when the primary tumor is very small (less than 1 millimeter thick) and has not spread to other parts of the body. Stage II cancer is when the primary tumor is larger (greater than 1 mm thick) and has not spread to other parts of the body. Stages 0 through II are therefore cancer *in situ*. Stage III cancer is when the cancer has spread to nearby lymph nodes and to nearby organs. Stage IV cancer is when the cancer has spread to distant organs in the body and is metastatic and inoperable. Another important stage is the recurrent stage, which is when cancer returns after treatment. It may come back in the same part of the body or in another part of the body. At this stage, the cancer is extremely difficult if not impossible to treat. If the cancer is untreatable, the patient is often given treatment that will help to relieve the discomfort and pain that metastatic cancer usually causes. More detailed staging systems can be found on the National Cancer Institute's Web site (http://www.cancer.gov). Finally, it is important to know that the specifics of cancer staging may change, since scientists are constantly finding out new information about a given cancer, requiring it to be recategorized.

SUMMARY

Cancer is a complex group of diseases. At the basic level, our genes are important in determining whether we have an increased chance (susceptibility) of developing cancer. Environmental factors, such as air pollutants or high-energy radiation, can greatly increase our chances of getting this disease. If the cancer is detected early and has not spread to other parts of the body (metastasis), there is a good chance that a person will survive the cancer; if it has metastasized, whether or not a person will respond to therapy is largely dependent on the type of cancer, but in general, advanced metastatic cancers are almost impossible to cure. This is why we all dread to hear the word "cancer." On a brighter note, however, at the end of 2006, the American Cancer Society reported that the number of cancer deaths has been decreasing. This has been attributed to better awareness of the body with regular medical check-ups that pick up early cancers that are more treatable. This is certainly the case for skin cancer, as we will see in the following chapters.

2

THE SKIN

KEY POINTS

- The skin is an organ with many specialized functions.

- It consists of three major layers—the epidermis, dermis, and hypodermis.

- The epidermis is a "stratified" epithelium with layers of specialized cell types.

- The skin contains stem cells, which give the skin its high regenerative properties.

What is the largest organ we have? Many people would say the liver, brain, or heart, but they would be wrong. An organ is defined as a collection of tissues that perform a particular function or set of functions. Therefore, the largest organ of the body is actually the skin, which makes up about one-third of a person's total body weight. Our skin covers our entire body, comes in various shades of color, and holds together all the components of our body in one compact form. The skin is also a highly versatile organ with various functions:

1. Barrier protection against environmental elements such as solar energy rays or radiation and the weather. It also offers protection against physical forces and chemical agents.

2. Immunological protection against harmful environmental pathogens, such as parasites, viruses, and bacteria. The skin contains immune cells—naturally occurring cells in the body that defend us against infection by organisms such as bacteria and viruses that try to penetrate the skin's surface.

3. Providing a water-impermeable barrier to prevent us from becoming waterlogged or dehydrated.

4. Thermoregulation. The skin has a subcutaneous fat layer that acts as insulation to prevent heat loss by the body. The skin also contains hair follicles that can trap heat or release heat from the skin. When the body overheats (during exercise, for example), it is rapidly cooled by perspiration (sweating): Sweat is released from pores in the skin and, as it evaporates at the surface, it cools the body down. Heat can also be released (dissipated) by the widening of blood vessels near the skin surface, which brings more of the warm blood to the skin surface so that the body's heat can evaporate into the surrounding cooler environment. This process is called vasodilation. On the other hand, if the body feels cold, the blood vessels in the skin can narrow by vasoconstriction, drawing the blood vessels away from the skin surface, thereby preventing the "warmth" in the blood from evaporating away from the skin surface.

5. Metabolism of vital nutrients for the body. The skin is a valuable source of vitamin D3 (cholecalciferol). The major function of vitamin D3 is to maintain normal blood levels of calcium and phosphorus, which is essential for normal bone and teeth development. Vitamin D3 is made from 7-dehydrocholesterol (a cholesterol-derived molecule) found at high levels in the epidermal layer of skin, specifically in the stratum basale and stratum spinosum. Ultraviolet radiation provides the energy for enzymes to convert 7-dehydrocholesterol into vitamin D3, which is then transported to the liver and kidney where it is converted into vitamin D, 1.25 dihydroxyvitamin D, which is important in regulating many biological processes, such as bone formation. It has also been suggested to prevent cancers such as prostate, breast, pancreatic, and colon cancer.

6. Neurosensory functions. The skin contains many sensory nerves that give us the sensation of pressure, pain, and temperature. The skin also contains nerves called proprioceptors, which tells us when we are being touched. Proprioreceptors are sensory nerves that detect motion or the position of the body that is being stimulated.

SKIN STRUCTURE

The skin is mainly divided three layers: the epidermis, dermis, and hypodermis. These different cellular layers are important for maintaining the skin's integrity (wholeness). The uppermost layer, the epidermis, is the translucent skin layer that we can see and is in direct contact with the environment. This layer is made up mainly of epithelial cells called keratinocytes, which mature (differentiate) into cells that will eventually form the intact and waterproof barrier of the skin. This process is also called **stratification**. Below the epidermis is the dermis, a relatively thick layer that consists of nerve endings, blood vessels, oil-containing sebaceous glands, and hair follicles. This layer also contains the proteins **collagen** and **elastin**, which allow the skin to be tough and elastic, respectively. The third and lowest layer in the skin is the subcutaneous layer, which is made up mainly of fat cells, but also contains the roots of hair follicles and blood vessels. This layer protects against cold and acts as a cushion against pressure, and also attaches the skin to the muscles and connective tissue lying below it.

THE EPIDERMIS

The epidermis is on average about 0.1 mm thick and contains no blood vessels. It is divided into four main layers: the stratum basale (basal layer), the stratum spinosum (spinous or prickle-cell layer), the stratum granulosum (granular layer), and the uppermost **stratum corneum** (surface layer). This last layer is the one that is in direct contact with the environment. Every day we shed many thousands of dead cells from our skin, which are replaced by keratinocyte cells from the lower layers of the epidermis that move upward and become cells that have specialized functions required to keep the skin intact and healthy. Our bodies reproduce a new epidermal layer approximately every 30 days. When damaged, the epidermis is capable of regenerating itself, generally without **scarring**. Thus, the epidermis has an incredible capacity to regenerate throughout our lifetime.

LAYERS OF THE EPIDERMIS

The stratum basale, or "basal layer," is the lowest epidermal layer and is separated from the lower dermal layer by the basement membrane—it

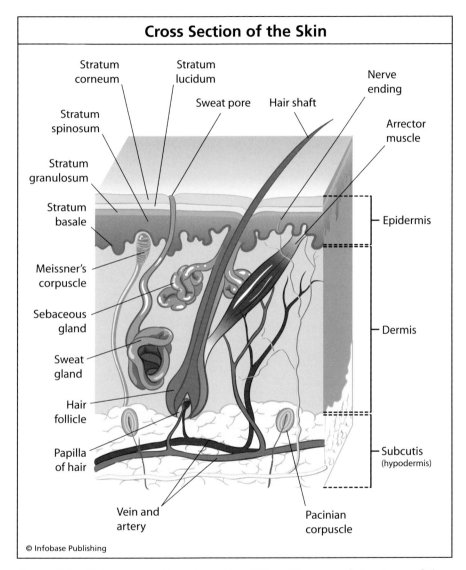

Cross Section of the Skin

Stratum corneum

Stratum lucidum

Stratum spinosum

Sweat pore

Hair shaft

Nerve ending

Arrector muscle

Stratum granulosum

Stratum basale

Epidermis

Meissner's corpuscle

Sebaceous gland

Dermis

Sweat gland

Hair follicle

Papilla of hair

Subcutis (hypodermis)

Vein and artery

Pacinian corpuscle

© Infobase Publishing

Figure 2.1 This cross section shows the different layers and structures of the skin.

is so called since it is at the "base" of the epidermis. The basal layer is responsible for the skin's remarkable capacity to regenerate because it contains the cells that give rise to all of the skin's epithelial cells. Basal

♦ **EPIDERMAL THICKNESS**

In most areas of the body, the epidermis is only 35 to 50 micrometers thick. (A micrometer is one-thousandth of a millimeter.) The palms and the soles are usually much thicker (up to several millimeters). This makes sense since there is a lot of wear and tear that happens to the hands and feet. In other areas, such as around the eye region, the epidermis is only 20 to 50 micrometers (0.02–0.05 millimeters) thick and is extremely sensitive to abrasion and irritating substances. The thin epidermis around the eye also contains many blood vessels that show through the epidermis. The appearance of "panda eyes"—dark under-eye shadows—and the "puffy eye" look is thought to be the result of less blood flow around the eye region and a buildup of **lymph** (caused by bad circulation) and is easily seen through the thin skin.

keratinocytes may divide to make more basal keratinocytes or they may undergo a maturation process known as **keratinization**, in which cells become more specialized to carry out their specific function. These specialized cells then make their way to the skin's surface.

The thin basal layer is made up of two main populations of basal keratinocytes: the skin **stem cells** and the **transiently amplifying cells**. Stem cells are immature, **undifferentiated** cells (i.e. immature cells that have yet to become a certain cell type). They have unlimited dividing capabilities and can generate many identical copies of themselves, thereby increasing the stem cell population, or they can give rise to the more differentiated transiently amplifying cells, These are cells that are

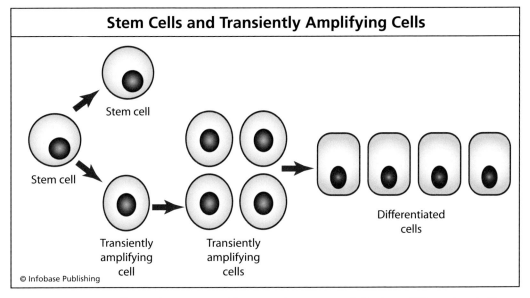

Figure 2.2   Stem cells are immature and have not become specialized, or differentiated. They can either give rise to more stem cells or create transiently amplifying cells, which divide for a short time until they become differentiated.

on the way to develop into a certain cell type, but are not yet mature. They divide for a short time and then differentiate into mature cells.

STEM CELLS IN THE SKIN

The definition of a stem cell is that it must have a) the capacity for self-renewal—it must be able to replace itself; b) a long shelf life to last a person's lifetime; c) a high proliferative potential—the capability to divide many times and generate many cells; and d) the ability to develop into many different cell types. Keratinocyte stem cells give rise to all the cell layers of the epidermis. A main source of stem cells has been found in a region lying next to the hair follicle called the **bulge**. These cells have the capacity to form new hair follicles and new epidermis. In areas of the body where there are no hair follicles, such as the palms of the hands, soles of the feet, and the lips, skin stem cells are believed to lie at the base of the undulating (wavy) ridges of the basal epidermal layer.

THE TRANSIENTLY AMPLIFYING CELLS OF THE BASAL EPIDERMIS

The other, more abundant type of basal keratinocyte is the transiently amplifying cell. This type of cell has a limited ability to divide. Once these cells have reached their dividing limit—predetermined by the

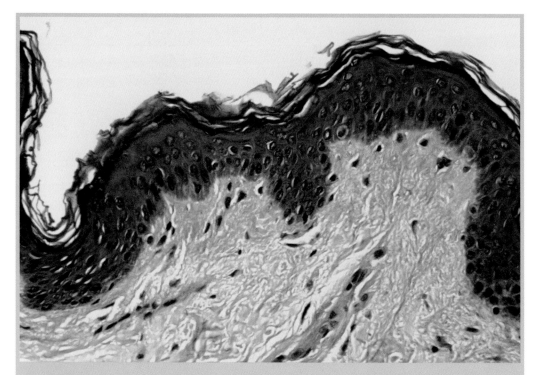

Figure 2.3 Photomicrograph of normal human skin, magnified 312.5 times. The epidermis, in darker pink, contains four types of distinct cells: keratinocytes, melanocytes, Merkel cells, and Langerhans cells. *(Jean Claude Revy – ISM/PhototakeUSA.com)*

genes, which sets an internal molecular timer—they begin to differentiate into more specialized cells of the epidermis and migrate upward toward the skin surface. It is thought that most skin cancers come from the basal layer of the epidermis and that some skin cancers may originate from the stem cell compartments of the epidermis and the hair follicle bulge region.

THE UPPER LAYERS OF THE EPIDERMIS: THE SQUAMOUS CELLS

The stratum spinosum and stratum granulosum layers are the next layers up from the basal layer. Cells from the basal layer begin to mature and migrate upward into the stratum spinulosum. These cells become cuboidal (oblong) in shape and are generally referred to as **squamous cells**. These cells make up the majority of human epidermal cells. Active protein synthesis occurs in stratum spinosum to produce proteins called **keratins**. These proteins clump together to form **tonofibrils**, which reach out in the cytoplasm to converge on the **desmosomes**, which are structures in the epidermal cell membranes that stick to other desmosomes on neighboring epidermal cells. Desmosomes give the squamous cells in this stratum spinosum their characteristic prickly or spiny appearance.

The stratum granulosum is typically one to three rows of flattened, squamous cells and is the highest layer in the epidermis where living cells are found. They accumulate keratohyalin granules, which contain high amounts of filaggrin, which binds keratin fibers together in epidermal cells. Keratohyalin granules give the cells of the stratum granulosum their grainy appearance: Their properties, along with the desmosomal connections form the waterproof, continuous barrier that prevents fluid loss from the body. The granules also contain fat

◆ STEM CELLS

There is a great deal of excitement in the scientific and medical worlds about the potential of stem cells to cure diseases that are currently not curable. The reason for this interest lies in the unique ability of stem cells to turn into different types of cells.

There are two main categories of stem cells: embryonic and adult stem cells. Embryonic stem cells are stem cells that are found exclusively in the early stage embryo (when the embryo is a ball of approximately a couple thousand cells). Embryonic stem cells can generate any cell in the body and are termed **totipotent**. Adult stem cells are found in "niches" in organs including the brain, intestine, breast, lungs, and hair follicles. These stem cells can only develop into certain cell types and so they are termed **pluripotent**.

There is controversy about using embryonic stem cells since these cells are taken from embryos that will not have the chance to develop into human beings. They are usually obtained from embryos that have been developed in a test-tube—this is called *in vitro* fertilization. It is done if a couple has difficulties in having a baby by normal ways. Many of the woman's eggs are fertilized *in vitro* to increase the chance of making viable embryos. Of these fertilized eggs, only two to three fertilized eggs are implanted each time into the woman's womb to develop into babies. Implanting too many fertilized eggs would cause complications

molecules called lipids that are thought to act as intercellular cement to hold the cells together to help prevent our skin from splitting. This layer also contains tonofibrils.

to the pregnant mother and to the unborn babies if too many of these eggs develop into babies in the womb. These leftover fertilized eggs are generally discarded by the clinics. Therefore, instead of wasting them, researchers and clinicians would like to use these "early stage" embryos to obtain embryonic stem cells to carry out research that may lead to new therapies to treat diseases, such as **neurodegenerative** (nerve-destroying) **diseases** like Parkinson's disease and motor neurone disease, which are characterized by the destruction of nerve cells in the brain and spinal cord. Heart disease, which afflicts millions of people around the world and is the number one killer in the Western world, is caused by damage to heart cells. This is another disease that might be cured if stem cells could generate new heart cells to replace the damaged and dying heart tissue.

Because of the controversy of using embryonic stem cells for therapies, however, many researchers are focusing on finding and manipulating adult stem cells (by adding genes or proteins, for example) to make them more like embryonic stem cells. Not enough is known, however, about what makes an embryonic stem cell so totipotent, so it is difficult to know what to add. If we know the location of the adult stem cells in every organ and are able to manipulate them, we may be able to treat a wide variety of diseases. So far, adult stem cells have been identified in the blood, central nervous system, liver, intestine, pancreas, hair follicles, and skin. These have the potential to develop into many cell types of that particular organ, but not into all cell types of the body.

In thicker areas of epidermis, such as the hands and soles of feet, there is normally a layer called the **stratum lucidum**, which represents the transition from the stratum granulosum to the stratum corneum. Cells in the stratum lucidum are already beginning to degenerate to develop into the next layer up, the stratum corneum. Since this layer is not found in thin skin, it is not considered a major epidermal layer.

As the cells begin to reach the outermost layer of the epidermis, the stratum corneum (also known as the **horny layer**), the dying cells become fully keratinized, begin to flatten out, and are fused together by lipids made by the stratum granulosum. This layer is mainly made up of dead cells that lack nuclei. The protein involucrin is produced by the stratum granulosum, and in the stratum corneum, it forms a thickened layer on the inner side of the **plasma membrane** of cells. Deeper cells in the stratum corneum retain their desmosomes and are essentially pushed upward to the skin surface by newly forming cells of the basal epidermis. It is thought that in cells of the corneal layer, **lysosomal enzymes** (enzymes that break down complex molecules) eventually cause the cells to start to die. Gradually, as they die and break apart, they slough away in a process called **desquamation**.

NONEPITHELIAL CELLS IN THE EPIDERMIS

There are multiple types of nonepithelial cells present in the epidermis.

Melanocytes

Also located in the basal layer of the interfollicular epidermis are the skin melanocytes. These cells produce the pigment melanin, which is the substance that gives our skin its color. The condition **albinism** in which affected people produce very little melanin gives them a characteristic appearance of extremely white skin, as well as white hair and red eyes. More importantly, melanin provides protection against ultraviolet radiation (UVR). Melanocytes make up 5 percent to 10 percent of the cells in the basal layer of the epidermis, with about 1,000 and 2,000 melanocytes

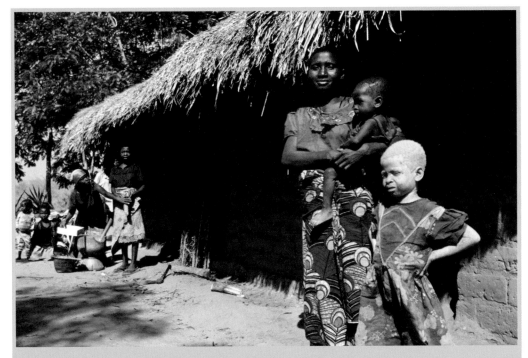

Figure 2.4   An African albino boy. *(BURGER/PHANIE/Photo Researchers, Inc.)*

per square millimeter of skin. Mature melanocytes form long dendritic (branch-like) projections that reach out along neighboring epidermal keratinocytes. Each melanocyte makes contact with about 30 to 40 keratinocytes. This interaction between the cells allows the melanocyte to transfer melanin through melanosomes (pigment-producing granules) to the keratinocytes. Once in a keratinocyte, melanin form caps around the nucleus to protect their DNA against the damaging effects of UVR. Melanin production is controlled by melanocyte-stimulating hormone produced in the pituitary gland, epidermal keratinocytes, Langerhans cells, and melanocytes. UVR can induce an increase in melanin production, resulting in tanning.

All human beings, regardless of race, have the same number of melanocytes. Therefore, it is not the quantity of melanocytes that determines
skin color but the number and arrangement of the melanosomes within
the keratinocytes. Melanosomes that grow together in benign clusters
are called **moles** or **nevi**. Moles generally grow or change slightly over
long periods of time and occasionally may acquire cancerous genetic
mutations resulting in melanoma.

Langerhans Cells

The Langerhans cells are immune cells that lie in the epidermis. They
function as local responders to skin infections, guarding against pathogens that might try to attack the skin. When they encounter an invading
pathogen, they leap into action by taking up the pathogen, processing
it and moving it to a nearby lymph node, where other immune cells,
such as white blood T cells, pick up the information about the would-be
invaders and mount an immune response against them.

Merkel Cells

Merkel cells are slow-acting **mechanoreceptors** in the basal layer of the
epidermis that sense touch and hair movement. They are neuroendocrine
in origin—that is, they originate from cells that had characteristics of both
the neural and endocrine systems. It is important to know about the origin
and characteristic of cell types since cancer treatments can be determined
by this. Merkel cells have the ability to develop into an aggressive cancer,
Merkel cell carcinoma, although the number of cases is extremely rare.

THE HAIR FOLLICLE

Hair is one of the most distinguishing features of a person. We have hair
follicles over most our body. On the head alone, there are more than

◆ SKIN COLOR

The melanocyte is responsible for producing the skin's pigment, melanin. There are two types of melanin: the brown-black eumelanin and the reddish phaeomelanin. Although all melanocytes produce both types of pigment, eumelanin is produced in greater amounts in the epidermis of people with dark skin and dark hair, while phaeomelanin is predominant in the epidermis of people with white skin and/or with red, blond or light brown hair. Once the melanin is produced by the melanocytes, it is packaged into melanosomes, which move along the melanocytes' branch-like projections, into the nearby epidermal keratinocyte cells. There, melanin provides protection against the sun's ultraviolet rays by absorbing them and stimulating DNA repair. The number of melanocytes is constant in all human skin types. In black skin, however, the melanosomes are larger than those in white skin, contain more melanin and are packaged as single units rather than as groups (as in white skin). This prevents them from degrading, thereby increasing the level of skin pigmentation that gives the appearance of dark skin. When we are exposed to UVR, production of both types of melanin increases; however, it is thought that the eumelanin is responsible for how deep in color the tan is.

100,000 hair follicles. These structures are derived from epidermal stem cells that lie in the region below the follicular epidermis, in a pocket known as the bulge, which is part of the basal epidermis known as the outer root sheath since it sheaths the hair root.

Each hair follicle goes through three phases. The first is called **anagen**, which is the active growth phase. The second is **catagen**, the phase in which part of the hair follicle degenerates, leading to the loss of the hair shaft while the remaining portion, the hair root, stays deep in the dermis and subcutaneous layer. This is why our hair falls out. The last phase is called **telogen**. This is the resting phase of the hair follicle cycle. The remaining hair follicle then enters the growth phase again when genetic and cellular signals from the base of the hair follicle signal to the hair follicle stem cells to initiate a new hair follicle: There is rapid cell proliferation of bulge stem cells to generate new hair. Each follicle is connected to a sebaceous gland, which releases the oily sebum that gives hair its glossy appearance. It has been suggested that some skin cancers may arise from these follicular stem cells.

THE DERMIS

The dermis is the thick layer of cells lying under the epidermis. It is responsible for supplying the epidermis and itself with nutrients and oxygen carried by the blood. The dermis is subdivided into two regions: the **papillary dermis** and the **reticular dermis**. The papillary dermis is so-called because of its fingerlike projections—*papillae*—that extend toward the epidermis and provide a strong connection between the two layers. It contains mainly cells called **fibroblasts** that secrete collagen, elastin, and other molecules that are needed for the support and elasticity of the skin. The thicker reticular layer contains denser, irregular, connective tissue (which is mainly collagen and elastin) and is also important for the overall strength and elasticity of the skin.

The dermis contains the **erector pili muscles**, which controls the orientation of the body hairs. When the muscles pull the hair erect, it gives the "goose bumps" or "goose flesh" look. It also contains apocrine (scent) glands, along with cells of the immune system and sebaceous glands. The cells in sebaceous glands—the **sebocytes**—produce and secrete sebum, the skin's natural oil. Cancer of the sebaceous gland can arise from sebocyte stem cells and is called sebaceous gland carcinoma. This type of cancer is extremely rare.

Also lying in the dermis are specialized neurons, which are required for skin sensitivity. These include: **Pacinian corpuscles**, which are **encapsulated** (enclosed by a protective coating or membrane) by mechanoreceptor (pressure receptor) nerves located deep in the skin that respond to heavy pressure; Meissner's corpuscles, which are also a type of mechanoreceptor located close to the skin surface and respond to light touch; Krause end bulbs, which detect cold temperature changes as well as touch and pressure; Ruffian end organs, which detect warm temperature changes as well as touch and pressure; and nerve endings that detect pain, which lie close to the dermal surface.

THE SUBCUTANEOUS LAYER

Below the dermis is the subcutaneous layer of the skin, which contains fat-filled adipose cells. The main functions of this layer are to act as insulation against heat loss from the body. It also provides an energy reserve, similar to the way hibernating animals store fat in their body for the winter when food may be limited. Hibernation is when animals slow down their metabolism, lower their body temperature and breathing rates, and gradually use up the body fat reserves stored during the warmer months, to survive the winter months.

The subcutaneous layer is loosely attached to connective tissue (tissue that supports or fastens together other body tissue or parts), which allows the skin to move relatively freely. The fat cells are arranged as lobules, which are separated by collagen fibers (protein fibers produced by skin cells that give the skin strength and resilience). In adults who have too much subcutaneous fat, the points at which the connective tissue links to the fat lobules has a pocked or rippled appearance, commonly called cellulite. The distribution of subcutaneous fat in the body differs between men and women. In women, more fat is stored in the buttocks and thighs, while in men, fat is stored in the abdominal wall, giving the characteristic "beer belly" appearance. The subcutaneous layer also houses the roots of hair follicles when they are in their growing phase and blood vessels that supply nutrients to the skin.

SUMMARY

The skin is a highly specialized and crucial organ that we cannot live without. It is also one of the first things we notice about a person. Just by looking at someone's skin we get a lot of information about the person's age, race, diet, and health. As with other organs in the body, the skin needs good maintenance and protection from the environment to keep it in good functional order. It is an organ that is very exposed to many environmental dangers, such as the sun's ultraviolet rays, which can often lead to cancer, as we will see in the following chapters.

3

THE BASICS OF SKIN CANCER

> **KEY POINTS**
>
> ♦ Skin cancer is the most common human cancer.
>
> ♦ The Caucasian population is most susceptible to developing skin cancer.
>
> ♦ There are two main groups: melanoma and nonmelanoma skin cancer.

At the end of 2006, U.S. first lady Laura Bush had a "troublesome patch" that was about the size of a nickel on her right shin, which would not heal. After consulting a doctor, the "patch" was promptly removed and histological analysis (looking at the cellular organization using a microscope) of the patch indicated that it was a skin tumor—a squamous cell carcinoma. Although Mrs. Bush had to wear a bandage to protect the region where the tumor was removed, she had no further complications. She will have to be carefully monitored for new skin cancers in the next five years, however, since there is an increased chance of developing another skin tumor if a person has already had one.

Skin cancer is the most common human cancer. At present, a cancer is termed "common" if there is annual incidence of 30,000 cases or more. One out of every three newly diagnosed cancers is a skin cancer and approximately one million new cases of skin cancer are diagnosed in the United States every year. Before the 1970s and 1980s, skin cancer used to mainly affect older people, especially men who worked outdoors. Indeed, approximately 40 to 50 percent of 65 year olds in the United States will develop at least one form of skin cancer. In recent years, however, there has been a steady increase in the number of younger people developing skin cancer. A reason for this is that more young people are exposing themselves to higher levels of ultraviolet radiation (UVR) due to the perception that a "healthy tan" makes a person more attractive. An Australian study carried out in the early 1990s by Ron Borland and his group at the University of Melbourne Centre for Behavioural Research in Cancer, Anti-Cancer Council of Victoria in Australia, involved about 200 14-year-old high school students. These students were shown pictures of models with varying degrees of suntan ("no tan," "light," "medium," and "dark tan") and with different attire ("swimwear" and "casual"). Male and female students who participated had to judge which models looked healthier and more attractive. The results indicated that high school students thought that the "medium tan" was the healthiest and most attractive, and "no tan" was perceived as both the unhealthiest and least attractive. Furthermore, darker tans were judged to be healthier and more attractive on male models, and models who wore swimwear. This study is a testimony to the notion that people like to be suntanned despite the well-documented dangers of developing skin cancer caused by increased exposure to UVR. A suntan occurs when the skin is exposed to more UVR than the pigment melanin can absorb and the skin becomes "sunburned." Still, people like to lie in the sun and use sunlamps and tanning beds, knowing full well that the process of tanning can cause skin damage and skin cancer.

MELANOMA AND NONMELANOMA SKIN CANCERS

Skin cancer is divided into two main groups: **melanoma** and nonmelanoma skin cancers (NMSC). Melanoma is a cancer of the pigment-producing cells, the melanocytes. Although melanoma is rare (4 percent of all skin cancers), it is the most aggressive and deadliest form of skin cancer, making up 80 percent of deaths due to skin cancer. For NMSC, there are two main types: basal cell carcinoma (BCC) and squamous cell carcinoma (SCC). BCC is the most common form of any cancer and affects approximately 800,000 Americans each year, accounting for about 80 percent of all skin cancers.

SCC makes up approximately 16 percent of all skin cancers. As mentioned earlier, first lady Laura Bush had this type of skin cancer. The numbers of cases of NMSC are probably much higher, however, since these cancers are generally treated in a private doctor's office and are never reported to the **cancer registry**. The cancer registry is a database of all reported cancer cases. It includes information about when they occurred, the type of cancer, and other information. In the United States, the annual **incidence** of NMSC—approximately one million cases—is higher than the incidence of all other types of cancer combined. Although the numbers of NMSC are staggering, both basal cell and squamous cell carcinomas have a better than 95 percent cure rate if they are detected and treated early.

ULTRAVIOLET RAYS ARE THE MAIN CAUSE OF SKIN CANCER

The sun emits solar energy rays that are essential for life on Earth. It provides daylight and warmth that allows vegetation to grow. It is composed of **infrared radiation**, which is the main **wavelength** (distance between repeating units of waves) that provides heat, visible light, and ultraviolet radiation (UVR). These wavelengths are part of the **electromagnetic spectrum**.

Ultraviolet radiation can be divided into UVA, UVB, and UVC radiation. UVB and UVC have higher energy rays (or wavelengths) than UVA. UVC is absorbed by the **ozone layer** of the atmosphere before it reaches Earth, so it poses no threat to our skin. UVB penetrates

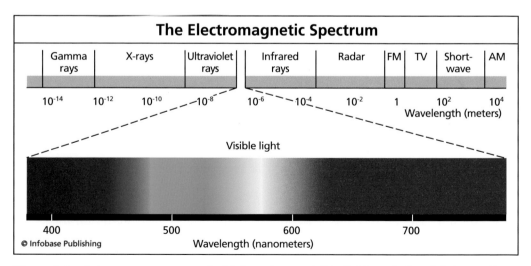

Figure 3.1   Solar rays are composed of infrared rays, visible light, and ultraviolet rays. Too much exposure to certain types of ultraviolet rays in sunlight can cause cancer.

only the upper layer of skin, the epidermis, and is responsible for the sunburn effect. It is the most cytotoxic (toxic to cells) wavelength of UVR. That is, it causes the most damage to our skin. UVA can penetrate deeper into the skin than UVB and is the main reason for premature aging and cellular damage, since it causes deeper connective tissue damage. It has been suggested that UVB causes BCC and SCC, while UVA is thought to cause melanoma.

Ultraviolet radiation can damage DNA directly in epidermal cells. It does this by "breaking" DNA and causing it to be altered to produce cyclobutane pyrimidine dimers (CPDs). This action by ultraviolet radiation gives rise to genes mutations, which can lead to skin cancer. In skin, (as in other organs) the *p53* gene is a major "protector" against DNA damage and is switched on when UVR causes DNA breakage, which is sensed by the cellular machinery. It codes for a protein that is important in regulating processes that are involved in "arresting" the damaged cell and/or making the damaged cell commit suicide (apoptosis). Like other genes, however, the *p53* gene itself is often mutated by UVR in skin cells. This probably increases the chance of a person developing skin cancer. Ultraviolet radiation can also suppress the immune function of skin: People who have a suppressed immune system (for example, organ transplant patients who need to take drugs to suppress their immune system to prevent organ rejection) have an increased chance of getting skin cancer.

The pattern of UVR exposure appears to be important in determining the type of skin cancer a person may develop. Intense, intermittent (off and on) exposure to sunlight is associated with a higher risk of developing BCC and melanoma. SCC, on the other hand, is thought to be more prevalent in people who are continuously exposed to the sun, such as outdoor workers.

OTHER CAUSES OF SKIN CANCER

Although exposure to ultraviolet radiation is the main cause of skin cancer, other factors can increase a person's susceptibility to skin cancer, such as a) exposure to ionizing radiation, such as X rays; b) exposure to arsenic (a naturally occurring element found in rocks and soil). Arsenic is commonly used as a commercial agricultural insecticide and poison; when combined with other elements and high doses it can cause skin cancer; c) heredity, such as when a genetic mutation inherited from a parent increases the chance that a person will develop skin cancer; d) organ transplantation—organ transplant recipients, who take immunosuppressive drugs to prevent organ rejection, are at a high risk of developing nonmelanoma skin cancer; e) viruses, such as the human papillomavirus (HPV), which is known to cause cervical cancer as well as a variety of skin **lesions**, including warts and SCC. HPV is thought to interact with carcinogens, such as ultraviolet radiation, to interrupt the skin's normal defenses against cellular damage, resulting in skin diseases.

RISK FACTORS FOR SKIN CANCER

Anyone can develop skin cancer. There are, however, some major factors that determine the likelihood of developing this disease, which are outlined below:

Ethnicity (Race) and Physical Characteristics

The group of people most at risk for skin cancer are Caucasians (white people of European descent), particularly redheaded, freckly, pale-skinned people of the Celtic (Irish and Scottish) populations. These people have type I and type II skin (Table 3.1). Type I people (redheads) never tan and always burn outdoors, turning a characteristic lobster-red color. They must always protect themselves from sunlight. People with type II skin (fair-haired types) tan very slightly and must also take precautions since they are also at high risk of sunburn and skin cancer. People with type III skin are average Caucasians who tan, but may also burn. Type IV skinned people are generally from the Mediterranean, Hispanic, and East Asian populations, while people with type V skin are of the Middle Eastern, Latino, Indian, and light-skinned black populations. Type VI skin—of dark-skinned black populations, such as Africans—rarely burn.

The color of a person's skin is therefore an obvious indicator of the likelihood of getting sunburn and subsequently developing skin cancer. It is not just skin color that is a factor, however, since some Asians have much paler skin than some Caucasians and still have less chance of getting skin cancer, so there is also a genetic component to the susceptibility to skin cancer.

Genetics

There are many diseases that develop as a result of an inherited mutation. If the mutation is in a gene that is normally important in controlling cell division and/or cell death, then the person who has the mutation may be more susceptible to developing cancer.

Youth

Young people have more sensitive skin than adults. Continuous exposure to ultraviolet radiation starting before the age of 18 can dramatically increase the chances of getting skin cancer, as well as **photoaging**. This permanent damage to the skin, caused by UVR, is seen in the form of wrinkles, age spots, blotchiness, freckles, and leathery, sagging skin that looks older than it really is.

Physical Location

People who live close to the equator are at a higher risk of developing skin cancer due to the higher ultraviolet radiation levels at this location. The equator is the closest point to the sun on Earth and is therefore exposed to the most intense UVR. **Indigenous** human populations that live at the equator generally have dark skin, which provides good protection. In the modern age in which we live, many fairer people travel and live in these areas and are at great risk of developing skin cancer. Although not on the equator but relatively close to it, Australia is a location that has a

TABLE 3.1 SKIN TYPE CATEGORIES		
SKIN TYPE	DESCRIPTION OF INDIVIDUAL	EFFECT OF UVR EXPOSURE ON SKIN TYPE
I	Bright white or pale skin; blue or green eyes; red hair; many freckles	Always burns outdoors and never tans
II	White skin; blue/gray eyes; blond or light brown hair; some freckles	Strong tendency to burn outdoors; tans minimally
III	Fair or light brown skin; brown eyes and hair	Burns moderately outdoors but always tans
IV	Light brown or olive skin; dark brown eyes and hair	Burns minimally outdoors and tans readily
V	Brown skin; dark brown hair and eyes	Rarely burns outdoors and tans easily
VI	Black skin; brown-black eyes and hair	Rarely burns outdoors

large number of fair-skinned individuals (due to mass immigration from Europe in the nineteenth and twentieth centuries), whose skin does not adequately protect them against the intense UVR. Hence, Australia has the highest incidence of skin cancer.

Personal Habits

A person who is exposed to sunlight for long periods of time is at higher risk of developing skin cancer than a person who stays indoors most of the time. This is because the damage caused by ultraviolet radiation is cumulative. That is, the amount of damage caused by UVR exposure "adds up" over time, so from 50 years old, after long-term or chronic exposure to the sun, the first skin cancers are seen.

THE INCREASE IN SKIN CANCER INCIDENCE

The number of new cases of skin cancer has risen dramatically over the past few decades. In the 1950s, people were not aware that excessive exposure to the sun was harmful. On the contrary, being out in the sun was thought to be beneficial. Therefore, many children would play outdoors without wearing any kind of protective clothing or sunscreen. This partly explains why cases of skin cancer have sharply increased in recent years, since these children who were chronically exposed to sunlight are now in their 50s and 60s and are developing their first skin cancers.

It is only in recent years that people have started to understand that chronic sun damage is not good if a person wants to stay younger-looking for longer and, more importantly, if one does not want to develop skin cancer. Australians in particular have to be careful about how much time they spend in the sun. Australia has the highest rate of skin cancer in the world because UV rays in Australia are higher than in

Europe and the United States. The Earth rotates about its axis in a way that brings Australia closer to the sun than Europe and the United States. This results in an increase of about 7 percent in UVR intensity from the sun. Also, Australia is close to the ozone hole, which lies above the ice landmass of Antarctica. Normally the ozone layer filters out much of the damaging UVR from the sun. Man-made air pollution such as car exhaust has contributed to the destruction of the ozone layer, making the hole bigger and exposing more of Australia to the harmful effects of the sun's rays. This means that because of Australia's location relative to

---

◆ VITAMIN D AND ULTRAVIOLET RADIATION

Vitamin D, or **calciferol**, is a fat-soluble hormone that is required for normal bone formation and to maintain normal levels of calcium and phosphorus in the blood. It is classified as a vitamin, but strictly speaking, it is not one since the skin can make it. The skin produces a significant proportion of bioactive ("having an effect on living tissue") vitamin D when UVB from sunlight reacts with the vitamin D **precursors** in the skin. In certain parts of the world, particularly in northern latitudes in the winter and in cultures that require people to completely cover their bodies from head to toe, vitamin D production in the skin may not be sufficient for normal body **homeostasis**. Therefore, people in these situations are encouraged to consume milk or commercial vitamin D supplements to boost their levels.

Vitamin D deficiency may lead to **rickets** in children and **osteo-malacia** ("adult rickets"), both of which are caused by a softening of

the sun and the hole in the ozone layer, Australians are exposed to up to 15 percent more UVR than Europeans. With a population roughly one tenth that of the United States's, there are about 280,000 skin cancers diagnosed each year in Australia, including 8,000 melanomas, and each year 1,200 Australians die from skin cancer. To combat the high incidence of cancer in Australia, there is now a drive for strong skin cancer prevention education.

It is not just Australia that is seeing a large increase in new skin cancer cases. Anywhere in the world that has a large Caucasian population

---

bones due to faulty mineralization—that is, the bones do not harden properly due to lack of mineral deposition. There are now data suggesting that vitamin D is also important in the prevention of many diseases, such as cancers, heart disease, depression, and diabetes. Some doctors have encouraged people to increase their exposure to sunlight to boost vitamin D production. This has raised concerns among cancer specialists who worry that people will "overexpose" themselves to the ultraviolet rays in sunlight, thus increasing their chances of developing skin cancer. Scientific studies indicate that a good amount of vitamin D is produced after only one minimal **erythemal dose** of UV exposure. An erythemal dose is the amount of radiation which, when absorbed by exposed skin, turns the skin temporarily red. This means that a fair-skinned adult produces enough vitamin D if he or she is in the sun for just 15 minutes two to three times a week. Longer exposures to the sun may be far more harmful than beneficial since ultraviolet radiation can also cause DNA damage.

◆ THE "HEALTHY" TAN

In ancient times and in some parts of the world today, society has associated beauty with having pale skin. Women used to go to extraordinary lengths to whiten their skin, such as using lead paint (in ancient Roman and Greek times), which can cause death by slow lead poisoning, and arsenic (in the tenth century), which also caused poisoning and death. Being "pale" was an indication that the person was of a higher class, while peasants often were tanned due to working in the field. Suntans became fashionable among the Caucasian population in the twentieth century due to general lifestyle changes (for example, vacationing in tropical climates and wearing more revealing clothes). The French fashion designer and style icon Coco Chanel, who was seen with a tan that she developed from her cruises from Paris to the South of France, helped to establish the tan as a symbol of the rich and famous.

Today a tan is still perceived as a sign of beauty in Western cultures (this is the opposite in Asian culture, where paleness is seen as more attractive), giving people a look of good health and youth. In reality, however, tanning actually increases the chances of getting premature wrinkles and skin cancer. Tanning is the protective response of the skin to ultraviolet radiation. When UVR reaches the skin, the skin pigment cells, or melanocytes, produce more melanin to absorb the UV rays and protect the skin's DNA from damage. This increased melanin production is what gives people a tanned appearance. If the amount of exposure to UVR is greater than the skin's ability to generate enough melanin, however, then protection from the harmful effects of UVR is compromised and DNA damage and sunburn occurs. The skin damage usually clears up within a few days with some skin peeling due to the killing of severely damaged skin cells; getting sunburned increases the chance of developing wrinkles and skin cancer due to the damage done to the remaining skin cells.

Indoor tanning beds were introduced in the 1970s, and by the 1980s artificial tanning was very popular in the United States. Early indoor tanning beds emitted the most damaging portions of the UV spectrum, UVC and UVB. In the 1970s, devices that emitted mainly UVA were developed, since UVA was considered the "safer" wavelength. Soon after, however, it became clear that UVA exposure caused the same problems as UVB— namely sunburn, wrinkles, and skin cancer. Also, the UVA-emitting devices were not as effective at inducing a tan. Since it took longer to get a tan from UVA-emitting devices, UVB-emitting devices came back into use. The devices used today contain a mixture of UVA and UVB, simulating the mixture found in the sun.

This notion that a tan symbolizes beauty, combined with the modern age of travel, led more and more people to head to sunnier climates or spend much of their time lying on artificial tanning beds, which allow them to maintain their suntan all year-round. The companies that make tanning beds have suggested that artificial tanning by this method is safe; however, this is not true since any darkening of the skin in response to ultraviolet radiation will cause DNA damage, regardless of whether the source of UVR is natural or artificial.

who regularly sun themselves will have seen an increase in the rate of new cases. In the common age of air travel, many more of us head off to warmer climates to sun ourselves each year. Also, it is not just the warmer climates that increase our chances of getting skin cancer. Outdoor pursuits such as skiing greatly increase our chance of getting skin damage and potentially developing skin cancer. This is because at the high elevations in which we go skiing, the air is thinner and therefore there are greater amounts of ultraviolet radiation. Also, snow and ice are highly reflective of UVR, which adds to our exposure.

Therefore, in the modern age, along with our genetics, our lifestyles and the environment can greatly increase our chances of developing skin cancer. Despite this, however, skin cancer is probably the most preventable of all the cancers and the most accessible for treatment.

SUMMARY

Skin cancer, the most common form of human cancer, can be divided into two types: melanoma and nonmelanoma. Many factors, such as genetics, age, and diet contribute to one's risk of developing skin cancer. The primary cause behind most skin cancers, however, is the exposure to ultraviolet radiation from the sun. Many cases of skin cancer can be prevented by avoiding excessive exposure to sunlight.

4

Basal Cell Carcinoma

KEY POINTS

- Basal cell carcinoma is the most common human cancer.

- It is an epithelial cancer that is thought to develop from the basal keratinocyte cells in the epidermis. It is slow growing and rarely metastasizes.

- Ultraviolet radiation and race are the main risk factors for developing basal cell carcinoma.

- The inherited form of basal cell carcinoma is known as basal cell nevus syndrome, which is caused by a genetic mutation in the gene *PATCHED1*.

- Basal cell carcinoma is highly treatable.

In the late 1990s, in an interview with Gary A. Taubes for the Howard Hughes Medical Institute, a young woman named Jenica Chekouras described how, at the age of six, she developed "weird moles" all over her body. These "moles" turned out to be basal cell carcinoma tumors and Jenica had the genetic disease basal cell nevus syndrome. In first grade, she told her classmates about her disease, who then told their parents. Ignorant about the disease, the children were told by their parents that they should stop playing with Jenica. That wasn't the worst of it, though. Numerous surgeries to remove these tumors followed throughout her teenage years and into adulthood. She will probably have to endure the tumor-removing surgeries for the rest of her life unless less invasive therapies are developed.

Basal cell carcinoma (BCC) has been described as far back as 4,000 years ago in ancient Egypt. Indeed, BCC-like tumor marks have been found on Egyptian mummies from those times. For centuries after, however, this cancer was categorized with a whole bunch of unrelated skin diseases, such as syphilis, lupus, and warts on the face—all "touch me not" skin diseases, which was the term used in the Latin version of a fifth century Bible. By the fourteenth century, the French physician Guy de Chauliac, arguably the most eminent of surgeons during the European Middle Ages and physician to Pope Clement VI, was the first to distinguish BCC from other types of facial ulcerated skin diseases. He also devised surgical equipment and techniques to remove such skin tumors, and perhaps a little more unconventional for today's medicine, he also suggested that BCC should be treated with topical remedies such as honey!

Basal cell carcinoma is the most common human cancer. One out of three new cancers diagnosed is a BCC, and every year in the United States, there are approximately 800,000 new cases. People of European descent have a greater risk of developing this cancer and more men than women are affected. BCC makes up 80 percent of all skin cancers. It is a slow-growing cancer that rarely metastasizes. As BCC tumors grow, however, they tend to invade into local tissues and cause much tissue destruction. This can result in severe physical disfigurement if left untreated. In extreme cases, if the tumor grows aggressively and is left untreated, the patient can lose an organ, such as an eye. In even more extreme cases, people have died due to complications associated with an aggressively growing BCC tumor. There was a case of a 53-year-old Caucasian man who went to his doctor to complain about a growth on his back, which had been growing for 15 years and was starting to cause him back pain. Not long after his initial visit to the doctor, he lost the ability to walk properly and had to seek emergency care. Body scans showed that the BCC tumor had grown and extended itself into his spinal cord, compressing it and damaging the spinal cord tissue. He had surgery to remove the tumor and damaged tissue, and a steel rod was placed into his spine. The man then developed an infection from the surgery and died. If the man had sought treatment earlier when the tumor was much smaller, it is unlikely that he would have died in this way.

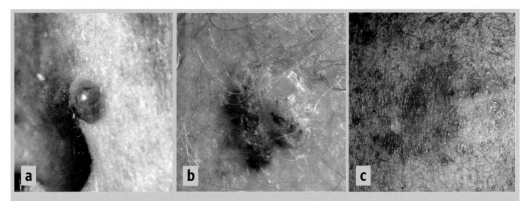

Figure 4.1 Various forms of basal cell carcinoma: a) nodular BCC, b) pigmented BCC, c) superficial BCC. (*Dr. Ken Greer/Visuals Unlimited; Biophoto Associates/Photo Researchers, Inc.; Dr. Ken Greer/Visuals Unlimited*)

Indeed, deaths from basal cell carcinoma are extremely rare, and most people will seek treatment when skin tumors are relatively small (less than half an inch in diameter). Former President Bill Clinton was diagnosed with a basal cell carcinoma on his back at the end of 2000, just before he left office. The BCC was promptly removed by surgery with no further complications.

BCC resembles the basal keratinocytes in the epidermis. BCC differs from many other cancers in that there does not appear to be a **precursor lesion**—an intermediate type of abnormal cell growth that will eventually turn into cancer—from which these tumors develop. In other words BCCs arise *de novo*. BCC tumors typically grow on the head, face, neck, hands, and arms. All of these areas of skin are chronically exposed to sunlight over the years. BCC tumors, however, can develop anywhere on the body.

In the majority of the population, BCC appears sporadically, and the average age of onset is approximately 60 years old. A small number of people, however—about 1 in 50,000—develop BCC from an early age (usually from the late teens) and generally have lots of tumors throughout their lifetime. This is because these people are genetically predisposed to this cancer, since they have inherited a germline mutation. The disease is called basal cell nevus syndrome (BCNS), nevoid basal cell carcinoma syndrome, or Gorlin Syndrome after the American physician, Robert James Gorlin, who was the first to describe this disease in the 1960s.

RISK FACTORS FOR BCC

Exposure to ultraviolet radiation is the main cause of all skin cancers. People with naturally red or blond hair, blue or green eyes, and light skin are most at risk of developing BCC. In contrast to squamous cell carcinoma, or SCC, the risk of developing BCC is significantly higher for people who have recreational exposure to the sun during childhood and adolescence. An example of recreational exposure is when we go to the beach or play in the park at the weekends. Other factors that are thought to increase our chances of getting BCC include exposure to certain chemicals such as arsenic and petroleum (crude oil) byproducts; exposure to ionizing radiation, such as X rays; chronic skin inflammation due to injury or an infection; medical conditions such as those that suppress the immune system over an extended period of time (for example, organ transplant patients develop more BCC than the general population); our behavior, such as how long we decide to stay in the sun, the type of clothing we wear; and our genetics.

THE GENE MUTATION THAT DIRECTLY CAUSES BCNS

In 1996, research groups headed by Ervin Epstein Jr., a dermatologist (a physician who specializes in diseases of the skin) at University of California, San Francisco, and Mathew Scott, a developmental biologist (a scientist who studies how a multicellular organism develops from its early immature form into an adult form) at Stanford University, discovered the gene that is the main causal factor in BCNS. People with this disease develop abnormally high numbers (tens to hundreds) of BCC tumors from an early age. The disease also ran in families, indicating that it was caused by inherited genetic mutation. Epstein's group and others had mapped the disease to a region of chromosome 9 in humans by comparing the DNA between affected family members to see whether they had the same genetic mutation. Scott's lab had identified the *patched* gene in fruit flies and mice. Mutations in the gene gave the embryonic fruit fly a "patchy" pattern in the bristles, hence the name *patched*. Scott's group found a similar gene sequence on chromosome 9 in humans and looked in the literature to see whether there were any diseases linked to this chromosomal region. Lo and behold, there were publications indicating that this region on human chromosome 9 was linked to BCNS. Scott contacted Epstein and told him: "I think we've got your gene." Working together, they found that mutations in the *PATCHED* gene were the probable cause of BCNS, and their discovery was published in the journal *Science* in June 1996. On that same day, Allen Bale of Yale University and an international team of collaborators published in the journal *Cell* that the *PATCHED* gene was involved in BCNS. They also identified *PATCHED* gene mutations in sporadic (spontaneously-arising) tumors. Therefore, the discovery of the gene mutation that causes BCNS and BCCs is shared mainly by the two teams. The gene was renamed *PATCHED1* when another *PATCHED* gene (*PATCHED2*) was identified a few years later.

THE HEDGEHOG PATHWAY

The *PATCHED1* gene normally makes a protein that normally prevents the activation of a cellular and biochemical pathway known as the **Hedgehog (HH) signaling pathway** (Figure 4.2). In this pathway, the Hedgehog protein is at the top of its cell "signaling network": In the absence of HH, the HH pathway is repressed by PATCHED protein. When Hedgehog protein is present, however, it prevents PATCHED function, which then turns on a cascade of cellular and biochemical processes, which results in the activation of specific genes that are essential for normal development. The HH pathway is "highly conserved" in evolution. That is, it is found in many diverse organisms, from flies to humans. The *Hedgehog* gene was initially identified in the fruit fly in the 1970s by Christiane Nüsslein-Volhard (a German biologist) and Eric

F. Wieschaus (an American biologist) at the European Molecular Biology Laboratory (EMBL) in Heidelberg, Germany. These developmental biologists carried out a huge gene mutation screening experiment in fruit flies to identify genes that were involved in the development of an embryo. In 1995, Nüsslein-Volhard and Wieschaus (along with an American biologist, Edward Lewis) won the Nobel Prize for their many remarkable discoveries. Mutations in the *Hedgehog* gene caused fruit fly larvae to have a stubby and "hairy" appearance due to the disruption of the pattern of the hair-like projections that are found on flies. Hence, the larvae looked like hedgehogs, so the gene that was responsible for this was named *Hedgehog*.

Hedgehog, or HH, protein is active in embryo development, where it is important in regulating the processes that tells a cell what to become.

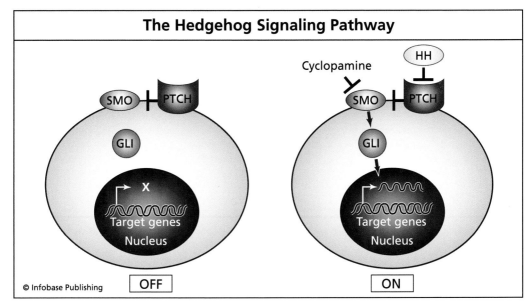

Figure 4.2   Abnormal activation of the cellular and biochemical pathway known as the Hedgehog signaling pathway causes several types of cancer, including basal cell carcinoma.

Also, signaling by HH tells cells to proliferate. In adults, Hedgehog signaling is generally not required in most cells and is switched off. However, it is active in regulating stem cell populations, such as in the hair follicle. In the past five years, scientists have discovered that abnormal activation of this pathway causes cancers other than BCC, including cancers of the brain, pancreas, lung, prostate, and intestine. Therefore, this "developmental" pathway initially found to be important for embryonic fly development is now known to be important in cancer development. Many scientists study this pathway in the hope of finding drugs that may block the activation of HH pathway-driven cancers such as BCC and medulloblastoma, a pediatric brain cancer.

BCC AND MUTATIONS IN THE HEDGEHOG PATHWAY

PATCHED1 gene mutations produce faulty PATCHED protein that can no longer keep the HH signaling pathway in check. Therefore, cells without this important tumor suppressor grow uncontrollably, become more genetically unstable, and become cancerous. People with BCNS have one defective copy and one normal copy of the *PATCHED1* gene. In other words, they are heterozygous for *PATCHED1*. Having just one functional copy of the *PATCHED1* gene does not mean that every skin cell will develop BCC. It just means that there is a greater chance of the skin cell becoming cancerous when exposed to an environmental carcinogen such as ultraviolet radiation. If this normal *PATCHED1* gene is hit, the cell will have no functional PATCHED1 protein to control the HH pathway. It is like removing the brakes of a car, except whereas a car eventually runs out of gas, runaway mutant skin cells continue to proliferate out of control, becoming even more unstable and have a good chance of developing a BCC tumor.

Since *PATCHED1* was linked to developing BCNS and BCC in 1996, many inherited and noninherited (sporadic) BCC tumors have been found to have *PATCHED1* mutations. In addition, mutations have been found in genes such as *SMOOTHENED (SMO)* that normally code for proteins that activate the HH pathway. These mutations change the code from making normal protein to making abnormal "super-active" proteins that cannot be switched off by the normal cellular regulators. In other words, these mutant proteins are "constitutively active" and always keep the HH pathway switched on, allowing cancer to develop. Their function is opposite to PATCHED1 function.

THE *P53* GENE AND BCC CARCINOGENESIS

The tumor suppressor gene *p53* has been called the "guardian of the genome." Mutations of *p53* are found in at least 50 percent of all BCC tumors that are analyzed. The *p53* gene codes for a protein that is important in regulating processes that mend DNA in cells that have been damaged—by UVR, for example. If the DNA is damaged beyond repair, *p53* sends out signals to tell the cell to kill itself. Therefore, *p53* is a very important gene required for protecting the genome, thus preventing the likelihood of cancer. The mutated *p53* gene, however, is often found in skin keratinocytes that are exposed to UVR. Because of these mutations in *p53*, the faulty p53 protein can no longer signal to the cells to mend its DNA, nor can it tell the cell to kill itself. Therefore, it is common to have patches of cells containing faulty *p53* genes and protein: these cells just divide and divide. It is not clear, however, whether the patches of mutant *p53* contribute to developing BCC.

◆ BASAL CELL NEVUS SYNDROME (BCNS) OR GORLIN SYNDROME

BCNS is an inherited condition in which afflicted individuals develop tens to hundreds of BCC tumors during their lives, starting in their early teens. It was first reported in 1894 by Adolf Jarisch, an Austrian dermatologist who described a patient with multiple BCC tumors, scoliosis (an abnormal curvature of the spine), and a learning disability. It wasn't until 1960 that the disease was properly characterized by the American physician Robert Gorlin, who described the full spectrum of malformations that people with the condition may develop. These malformations include defects of the eyes, nervous system, endocrine glands, bones, and skin. Children with BCNS have a characteristic appearance, with wide-set eyes; a broad-bridged nose; a heavy ridge over the eyes; a "unibrow" (single continuous eyebrow); and a protruding jaw. Perhaps the most striking abnormality seen in the teen years is the appearance of multiple BCC tumors, which frequently form around the eyes, upper lip, and cheekbones. Some 3 to 5 percent of children with BCNS develop medulloblastoma, (a common form of childhood brain cancer), and 25 to 50 percent of women with BCNS develop ovarian fibromas (benign tumors of the ovary). BCNS is inherited as an autosomal dominant disease—that is, an affected person only needs to inherit one faulty copy of the *PATCHED1* gene to develop the disease. People with this disease have to have numerous surgeries throughout their lifetime to remove the tumors and to correct some of the defects they develop.

CLASSIFICATION OF BCC SUBTYPES

BCCs come in different shapes and forms. These are classified depending on their **histology** and clinical behavior (i.e., the way the tumors acts in the tissue or organ). *Nodular* BCCs are the most common subtype of BCC. They account for 45 to 60 percent of all BCCs, and are frequently found on the head, neck, and upper back. They have a "pearly" appearance and can resemble waxy papules (small, solid, and usually conical elevations of the skin) with a central depression. Nodular BCC tumors may vary substantially since they can be ulcerated (a breakage in the skin), bleeding, crusted, or translucent. *Cystic* BCCs are uncommon variants of nodular BCCs and are sometimes difficult to distinguish from nodular BCCs. They may appear as translucent blue-gray, cyst-like tumors in which the center is filled with a gelatin-like substance, mucin (a cyst is a fluid-filled mass that is usually benign). *Pigmented* BCCs have features similar to those of nodular BCCs, but they also contain increased brown or black pigment. These tumors make up 1 to 2 percent of all BCCs and are seen more commonly in darker-skinned people, including Hispanics and Asians. A history of arsenic ingestion is also associated with pigmented BCCs. *Superficial* BCCs make up 15 to 30 percent of all BCCs and are the least aggressive since they don't often invade the underlying tissues. They can be scaly, dry, round, or oval patches that are pink to reddish-brown in color, often with central clearing (i.e., clear of tissue) and with a raised border. Superficial BCCs are common on the trunk and extremities, and are sometimes confused with other skin diseases such as psoriasis (a noncontagious inflammatory skin disease characterized by recurring reddish patches covered with silvery scales) or eczema (a common itchy, painful skin condition that is caused by contact with allergens). Superficial BCCs progress slowly and do not change in appearance. Exposure to arsenic may result in many of these BBC subtypes.

Aggressive BCCs are of the micronodular, infiltrative, morpheaform, and mixed variants. Patients younger than age 35 tend to have the more aggressive forms of BCCs. Micronodular BCCs appear similar to nodular BCCs but they are less prone to ulceration and look yellow-white when stretched. They have well-defined borders and are firm when you press down on them. Morpheaform and infiltrating BCCs make up 4 to 17 percent of all BCCs. They have a scar-like appearance, which is caused by tumor cells inducing the underlying dermal fibroblasts to proliferate and increase its collagen production. These types of BCC do not ulcerate, bleed, or crust, and may have undefined borders.

Trichoepithelioma is a BCC-like tumor that occurs spontaneously, or as an inherited autosomal dominant disease called multiple familial trichoepithelioma. These are small, benign, rare tumors that arise on the face after puberty (in early adulthood). They are thought to come from the basal keratinocyte layer in the hair follicle. There are three types of trichoepithelioma: solitary (single tumor), multiple (many tumors), and desmoplastic (whitish, hard nodules with a central depression, characterized by basaloid or basal keratinocyte-like cells and epidermal cysts infiltrating the stroma (fibrous connective tissue). Trichoepitheliomas are often confused with BCC because of their firm, rounded, and shiny appearance; however, trichoepitheliomas appear yellow, pink, brown, or blue. They usually increase in number with age, occurring on the cheeks, eyelids, and around the nose.

DIAGNOSIS OF BCCS

Any abnormal-looking skin growth should be examined by a dermatologist or a dermopathologist, who will carry out a biopsy under local
anesthetic to check whether the growth is cancerous. The biopsy
will then be looked at using a microscope to see what tumor type
it is. There are several different types of skin biopsy. Incisional and
excisional biopsies are done to see how far down into the skin a BCC
tumor has invaded. An incisional biopsy is when part of the tumor is
removed, while an excisional biopsy removes the *entire* tumor. Both
types of biopsies are done with a scalpel, and the skin around the
tumor is anesthetized before the biopsy. A shave biopsy is done if the
skin tumor is thought to only affect the epidermis and dermis. The
skin area is anesthetized and the growth is "shaved off" with a scalpel
or razor blade. This biopsy is useful to look at the many types of skin
diseases and for removing benign moles. In a punch biopsy, a "full
thickness" of the skin is removed. Once the skin is anesthetized, the
doctor rotates a tool that works like a miniature cookie cutter on the
surface of the skin. It cuts through all the layers of the skin and brings
up a sample of tissue.

If the tumor is suspected to be a BCC, the whole tumor has to be
removed. The treatments for BCC tend to be fairly straightforward and
successful.

STANDARD TREATMENTS OF BCCS

Generally, treatment for most benign skin cancers is carried out by
a dermatologist. In more complicated cases, a plastic surgeon and a
clinical oncologist (cancer specialist) may also be involved. The plastic

surgeon reconstructs the wounded site to minimize scarring, and the oncologist "grades" the tumor. The choice of treatment is based on the type, size, location, and depth of penetration of the tumor, as well as the patient's age and general state of health.

Simple Excision

With simple excision, tumors are cut out with a scalpel and a sample is sent off to a laboratory to undergo tumor margin evaluation. This process involves looking at the sample under a microscope to check whether the whole tumor has been removed. Doctors or lab technicians can tell by looking for the cellular boundaries (margins) of the tumor, which look different from normal skin cells. Tumor recurrence (when a tumor comes back) is common with this procedure, since only a small fraction of the total tumor is analyzed and is therefore not an accurate assessment. Simple excision surgery, however, is much cheaper, simpler and quicker to do than Mohs Micrographic Surgery.

Mohs Micrographic Surgery

This highly effective treatment is named after Dr. Frederic E. Mohs, who invented it in 1936 at the University of Wisconsin. It involves removing the visible tumor with a curette (a spoon-shaped surgical instrument) or scalpel and then removing thin layers of the remaining surrounding skin, one layer at a time. Each layer is checked under a microscope, and the procedure is repeated until the last layer viewed is cancer-free. This technique saves the greatest amount of healthy tissue and has the highest five-year cure rate for both primary (96 percent) and recurrent (90 percent) tumors. (A "five-year cure rate" describes the percentage of patients who have lived at least five years after their cancer is diagnosed without the cancer returning.) Mohs micrographic surgery is often used for tumors that have recurred or tumors that are in places such as the head, neck, hands, and feet to lessen the chances of the tumor recurring. It is also used for tumors with poorly defined clinical borders (not "well-contained") to increase the chances of removing as much of the tumor cells as possible.

Curettage and Electrodesiccation

This treatment involves scraping or scooping out the visible tumor cells with a curette (curettage) and drying out the tumor site with a high-frequency electric current applied with a needle-shaped electrode (**electrodessication**). This procedure is quick but requires local anesthesia and must be repeated a few times to make sure that all cancer cells have been eliminated. Small tumors (2–5 mm in diameter) have a 15 percent recurrence rate after this treatment, but with large tumors (larger than 3 cm in diameter), a 50 percent recurrence rate is expected within five years.

Cryosurgery

This treatment involves "freezing off" the tumor with liquid nitrogen, which is applied with a cotton-tipped applicator or spray. Liquid nitrogen is so cold that it causes the tissue to blister or to become crusted and then fall off. The treatment does not involve any cutting or anesthesia, although there is temporary redness and swelling after the surgery. Cryosurgery is used for patients with small, well-circumscribed primary tumors, and is especially useful for patients with other medical conditions, such as a bleeding disorder, that make other types of surgery impossible. Also, cryosurgery can be used to remove multiple tumors relatively easily. A disadvantage of cryosurgery is that treated tumor regions are left with permanent pigment loss, scarring, and/or exude necrotic material. Necrosis is the process by which cells die in response to disease or injury, expelling their damaged cellular contents onto neighboring cells and causing inflammation.

Radiation Therapy

This treatment involves directing X ray beams at a tumor to destroy it. It is used for tumors that recur and for elderly patients who are in poor health. As with cryosurgery, total destruction with radiation therapy requires several treatments a week for a few weeks. This treatment, however, produces less scarring and loss of pigment than cryosurgery does. It is commonly used for recurring tumors that arise after the surgical removal of the primary tumor. Radiation therapy is not used for patients with xeroderma pigmentosum (a genetic disorder that affects DNA repair) or for BCNS patients, since X rays induce more skin tumors in these people.

Carbon Dioxide Laser Surgery

This is most frequently used for BCCs that have not infiltrated the dermis. It is used if the patient is prone to bleeding due to a clotting defect, since this treatment does not cause bleeding.

Topical Fluorouracil (5-FU) Therapy

This is useful in the management of superficial BCCs in some patients. Patients apply the cream to their skin. With this treatment, patients require long-term monitoring, since portions of the tumor may be deep in the follicular region of skin and escape treatment, resulting in tumor recurrence.

Photodynamic Therapy (PTD)

This therapy uses topical photosensitizing (light-sensitive) drugs, such as 5-aminolevulinic acid (5-ALA), which are applied directly to the BCCs before those medicated areas are "activated" by a strong light. The activation of the photosensitizing drug by light causes the formation of cytotoxic chemicals that then destroy the tumor. It is used for superficial BCC tumors.

Interferon Alpha (IFN-α) Therapy

This therapy uses the IFN-α protein, which is produced naturally in the body to fight infectious agents. It is a relatively new treatment that has been shown to have some effect against BCCs.

Post-Treatment Care

Once a person has been treated for BCC, he or she is usually examined every six months to a year to check for new or recurrent tumors. It has been found that 36 percent of patients who develop a primary BCC will develop a second primary BCC within the next five years. Early detection of the tumor is desirable to prevent the development of a more aggressive, harder-to-treat tumor. Also, a person who has had a BCC is more likely to develop the other forms of skin cancer, such as squamous cell carcinoma and melanoma, since having one skin cancer is thought to sensitize the surrounding skin region to developing new cancers.

METASTATIC DISEASE

In extremely rare cases, BCC may become metastatic cancer. Metastatic basal cell carcinoma (MBCC) is a very rare cancer, making up approximately 0.03 percent of all BCCs, and it behaves like other types of metastatic cancers in that it is highly aggressive and very hard to cure. Men are twice as likely as women to develop this aggressive disease. The average age of onset is 45 to 59 years. MBCCs are thought to arise from long-standing, large BCCs that persist even after several attempts to remove them. Nearly 85 percent of MBCCs develop in the head and neck region and then spread, initially as BCC deposits, to nearby lymph nodes and then to distant lymph nodes. Finally, they move through the bloodstream to the lungs, bones, and other areas of the skin.

Similar to other metastatic cancers, MBCCs can be very aggressive and are highly resistant to conventional therapies such as surgery, radiation therapy, and **chemotherapy**. **Palliative care** (treatment that provides **symptom** relief but not a cure) may be given to reduce pain from bone metastases. Most patients have a survival time of 10 to 14 months after diagnosis, and only about 10 percent of MBCC patients are still alive after five years. Similar to other metastatic cancers, MBCC may occur years after the initial diagnosis and seemingly successful treatment.

PREVENTION OF BCC

The best way for most people to prevent BCC and other skin cancers is to avoid overexposure to ultraviolet radiation. People with the inherited disease BCNS will likely develop many BCCs irrespective of whether they are exposed to UVR, but they still need to avoid direct sunlight since exposure often makes their condition worse. In addition, adults with BCNS have a 50 percent chance of passing the disease on to their children, so genetic counseling may be useful. It is now possible to test during early pregnancy for the mutation in the *PATCHED1* gene that causes the disease.

FUTURE DEVELOPMENTS

There is a lot of research into developing preventive treatments that can be used effectively to prevent BCC development in people who are at high risk to develop many tumors. Since most sporadic and inherited BCCs are thought to be due to the dysregulation (abnormal regulation) of the Hedgehog signaling pathway, there are many attempts to target this pathway therapeutically with "small molecule" drugs. A naturally occurring small molecule inhibitor of the HH pathway called

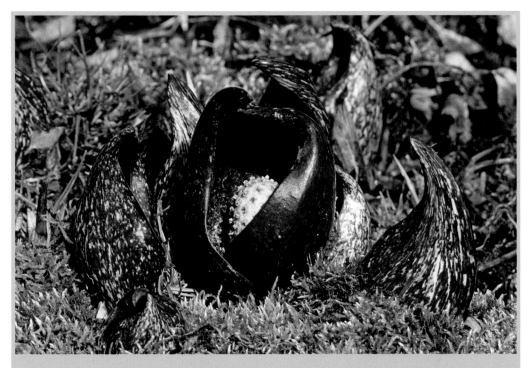

Figure 4.3 If eaten by a pregnant sheep, this skunk cabbage—which contains cyclopamine—may cause cyclopia in her young. (*Dick Poe/Visuals Unlimited*)

cyclopamine was identified in skunk cabbage, a plant that grows in the alpine meadows of the Rocky Mountains. Pregnant sheep that ate skunk cabbage gave birth to lambs with severe neurological damage including cyclopia—the fusion of the two eyes in the center of the face. From experimental animal studies done in the laboratory, this cyclopia was known to be caused by the inhibition of the HH pathway. Cyclopamine did not have any adverse effects on the adult sheep that ate the cabbage. Therefore, many researchers have suggested that making anti-cancer drugs that may mimic (copy) cyclopamine could specifically target cancers that are "driven" by increased HH signaling.

Indeed, in **murine** models of "Hedgehog pathway-driven" cancers, such as BCC and medulloblastoma, some cyclopamine-like molecules have shown good effectiveness against tumor growth. Properly controlled human trials are now required to test whether these drugs are actually effective in human subjects such as patients with BCNS.

Another potentially promising treatment for BCC chemoprevention is a topical retinoid (a synthetic vitamin A-related compound) called tazarotene (Tazorac). It is already approved by the Food and Drug Administration (FDA) for treating other skin conditions such as photoaging, psoriasis, and **acne**. Ervin Epstein Jr. (one of the researchers who identified *PATCHED1* as the gene mutation causing BCNS) and his lab are working on a carefully controlled human trial with BCNS patients to see whether tazarotene can prevent BCC from developing in these patients. His lab has already shown that tazarotene helped prevent BCC **carcinogenesis** in a murine model of the cancer. If it works in this human trial, other BCNS patients and even those patients who don't have the inherited disease but develop lots of BCCs will be able to rub in the cream just like a sunscreen.

SUMMARY

Basal cell carcinoma is the most common cancer in humans, but it is also one of the least dangerous of all cancers. It is a preventable cancer for most people and poses no real threat to human life. Since it is by far the most common cancer, however, the treatments and therapies needed to manage it create a huge financial and time-consuming burden on health services. Therefore, educating people about skin cancer prevention and looking for cheaper, less laborious alternatives to current therapies are probably the most effective ways to deal with this cancer. Education is the approach being taken in Australia, which has the highest incidence of BCC in the world. Developing BCC is not good news, but it is probably the best cancer to be diagnosed with since, for most people, BCC is easily detected, easily treated, and it rarely metastasizes.

5

SQUAMOUS CELL CARCINOMA

> **KEY POINTS**
>
> - Squamous cell carcinoma of the skin (SCC) is the second most common cancer.
>
> - Squamous cell carcinoma develops from squamous cells in the spinous layer of the epidermis.
>
> - Unlike BCC, SCC can arise from a noncancerous precursor growth.
>
> - SCC has the potential to metastasize; however, most SCCs do not.
>
> - Treatments for SCCs that have not metastasized are similar to those for BCC.
>
> - Treatments for metastatic SCCs are similar to those for other metastatic cancers.

In 1775, Sir Percival Pott, an English surgeon working in London, noticed that in chimney sweepers there was a high incidence of skin cancer of the squamous cell type (that is, SCC) on the scrotum (the bag of skin and muscle containing the testicles). Chimney sweeping involved repeated exposure to the soot produced by burning coal, and Sir Pott realized that the prevalence of this cancer in chimney sweepers was most likely due to "a lodgement of soot in the rugae (wrinkles) of the scrotum." We now know that chimney coal tar soot contains a substantial amount of carcinogens that can cause SCC. In Pott's time, however, the link of coal tar soot to SCC in chimney sweepers was the first time that an environmental agent and occupation had been directly linked to causing a cancer.

Squamous cell carcinoma of the skin is the second most common skin cancer, after basal cell carcinoma. It affects approximately 200,000 Americans each year. Like BCC, SCC of the skin is more prevalent among people of European ancestry, with a higher incidence in men than women. It is more common than BCC among African-American and Asian populations.

SCC develops from the squamous epidermis, which makes up most of the upper layers of skin. **Squamous epithelium** can be found in other parts of the body, such as the mucous membranes that line the respiratory and gastrointestinal tracts. The cutaneous form, however, is the most common type of SCC. As with BCC, ultraviolet radiation plays a major part in the development of SCC. Tumors develop mainly on areas of the skin that have been exposed to the sun. The physical distribution for BCCs and SCCs, however, is different on the body. SCCs are most common on areas of high ultraviolet radiation exposure (like the face) and BCCs are more common on areas of moderate UVR exposure, such as the upper trunk in men and women and the lower leg in women. It is thought that there is a linear relationship between sun exposure and the development of SCC—that is, the more sunlight we are exposed to, the greater the likelihood that we will develop SCC.

SCC is more dangerous than BCC since it is more likely to metastasize. The rate of malignant conversion from a nonmetastatic to a metastatic SCC is about 2 percent. SCC metastases most often develop on sites of chronic (long-lasting and recurrent) skin inflammation, or on mucous membranes and the lips. SCCs can develop from a precancerous lesion called **actinic keratosis** (unlike BCCs); however, some SCCs can arise without going through the precancerous stage (in other words, they arise *de novo*, like BCCs).

If a person is diagnosed with a SCC, the tumor is always removed since it has the potential to penetrate deep into the underlying tissues and destroy nearby tissue, and it has the potential to metastasize.

RISK FACTORS

Many of the risk factors for developing SCC overlap greatly with those for developing BCCs. As with BCC and melanoma, chronic exposure to UVR causes most cases of SCC. Tumors appear most frequently on sun-exposed parts of the body, such as the face, neck, bald scalp, hands, shoulders, arms, and back. The rim of the ear and the lower lip are especially vulnerable. People who are constantly exposed to the sun or artificial UVR for long periods of time are more at risk for developing this type of skin cancer than BCCs and melanoma, which are more common in people who have had only recreational exposure to the sun.

Ionizing radiation is also an SCC risk factor. In the early twentieth century, the link between this form of radiation and SCC carcinogenesis was established when SCCs were commonly found on the hands of experimental **radiologists**, due to their use of X rays, radium (a rare, brilliant white, luminescent, highly radioactive metallic element found in very small amounts in uranium ores), and radioactive isotopes (a form of an element with an unstable nucleus that "stabilizes" itself by emitting ionizing radiation). Exposure to these high-energy forms of radiation directly causes DNA damage, which can lead to cancer due to the accumulation of gene mutations even after body has "repaired" the DNA.

Exposure to toxic chemicals can also cause SCC. For example, arsenic ingestion results in development of multiple areas of SCC on the trunk and limbs some years after exposure (arsenic also causes white marks and scaly lesions on the palms and soles, called arsenical keratoses). Polycyclic aromatic hydrocarbons, which are made from the combustion and distillation of carbon compounds such as coal tar and cutting oils, can also cause SCC (as Sir Percival Pott alluded to in 1775). SCCs are commonly found on areas of skin with chronic inflammation, such as burns, scars, and long-standing sores. For unknown reasons, individuals of African descent are more likely to develop SCC than BCC, and they usually develop on the sites where inflammatory skin conditions or burn injuries have previously occurred. Immunosuppression is also a big risk factor for developing SCC. People who have had organ transplants are required to take immunosuppressive drugs to suppress the immune system over an extended period of time. These drugs prevent their body from rejecting the new organ; however, there is sharp increase the incidence of SCC in these patients. Also, people with a compromised immune system, such as patients with acquired immunodeficiency syndrome (AIDS) or blood disorders are also more susceptible to developing SCC. Viruses can also cause SCC. The human papillomavirus, or HPV, is known to cause cervical cancer in women. Recently, it has also been linked to the development of cutaneous SCC, since HPV had been found in 80 percent of the SCC tumors in patients who have received an organ transplant and in 30 percent of SCC tumors in people with a normal immune function.

Also, a person's history of skin cancer is also a high risk factor since there is a greater chance of developing skin cancer if he or she has already had already had one.

PRECURSORS OF SCC

Unlike BCC, some SCC tumors develop from precursor lesions, which may develop into SCC if not treated. These usually develop on skin with extensive sun damage. Actinic keratosis (AK) is a precancerous lesion that is thought to be the earliest form of SCC. It appears as a rough, scaly, slightly raised growth, ranging in color from brown to red and growing up to one inch (2.5 cm) in diameter. As with all other skin cancers,

---

◆ SCC AND TANNING: LESSONS FROM THE MOUSE

SCCs are commonly seen in outdoor workers, who are generally men. Today, however, SCCs affect more and more people, particularly young women who visit indoor tanning salons year-round to maintain a constant tan. Scientific experiments in which mice were exposed to ultraviolet light in many small doses—designed to simulate what indoor tanners might receive—showed that the mice developed more SCCs than they did when the same amount of ultraviolet radiation was delivered in a few big doses that resulted in sunburns. This suggests that tanning, rather than burning, may be more relevant for the induction of SCCs.

people with fair skin who sunburn easily and tan poorly, as well as those whose occupations or hobbies lead to excessive sun exposure, are most at risk of developing AK. It is suggested that between 1 percent and 20 percent of all AKs develop into SCC and that 60 percent of predisposed people over the age of 40 have at least one AK. Actinic chelitis (AC) is a type of AK that occurs on the lips (chelitis indicates that lesion on the lip). AC causes the lips to become dry, cracked, scaly, and pale or white. It mainly affects the lower lip, which typically receives more sun exposure than the upper lip.

Leukoplakias are white patches or plaques that are commonly found on the epithelium of the tongue or inside the mouth. It affects less than 1 percent of the population, and is most common in adults ages 50 to 70. Although the cause is unknown, tobacco use and chronic irritation have been linked to this disease, and sun damage can lead it to develop on the lips. Leukoplakia has the potential to develop into SCC.

SCC *IN SITU*: THE PRIMARY CANCER

Bowen's disease is considered a superficial SCC that has not yet spread—a SCC *in situ*. It is slow-growing and appears as a persistent, red-brown, scaly patch that may resemble psoriasis or eczema. It can appear anywhere on the skin but is most common on the head, the neck and the lower leg. If untreated, a Bowen's disease lesion may invade deeper structures and form a malignant SCC.

Carcinoma cuniculatum is a rare type of low-grade, invasive SCC also known as verrucous carcinoma. It is a slow-growing tumor with a hard, horny surface and is generally found on the sole of the foot. The exact pathogenesis (the mechanism by which a factor causes disease) of this

---

♦ ARSENIC AND SKIN CANCER

In the past, arsenic has been used in beauty products and in medications (to treat syphilis, for example). Today, high levels of arsenic can be found in tainted wine, metal ores, insecticides, and unprocessed well water. In many developing countries around the world, people get their drinking water from underground sources, often from simple hand-pumped tube wells, since surface water supplies are generally polluted. Many of these water sources have high levels of arsenic. This is causing a global epidemic of arsenic poisoning, with hundreds of millions of people thought to be at serious risk. Arsenic exposure results in invasive tumors and **carcinoma in situ** on the skin, whether or not the skin is exposed to the sun, as well as arsenical keratoses on the palms and sole, and liver cancer. Although arsenic is known to cause certain cancers, however, there is mounting scientific evidence that it may inhibit the development of other cancers.

---

cancer is not known, but it is thought to develop from a wart and has been linked to HPV infection and chemical-induced carcinogenesis.

Keratoacanthoma is a rapidly developing skin tumor that develops from a hair follicle and looks similar to SCC under the microscope. It disappears on its own accord, however, usually leaving a scar. Some clinicians believe it to be an unusual form of SCC. It appears as a hard, round papule that enlarges rapidly and becomes filled in keratin in the center to form a crusty covering. Keratoacanthoma tumors occur on their own or as multiple clusters on sun-exposed areas and mainly affect white males. An "eruptive" form of this tumor usually affects males and

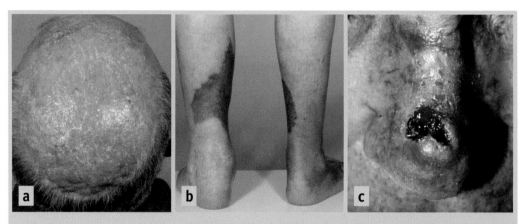

Figure 5.1 Various forms of squamous cell carcinoma: a) actinic keratoses, b) Bowen's disease, c) metastatic SCC. (*Bart's Medical Library/PhototakeUSA. com; National Cancer Institute/U.S. National Institutes of Health*)

females equally and often occurs in immunosuppressed patients, at the site of skin injury. It is sometimes associated with HPV infection.

APPEARANCE OF SCC

Like BCCs, SCCs come in various shapes and sizes (Figure 5.1a–c). In contrast to BCCs, however, many SCCs have a crusty, irregular appearance and may be observed as:

- a wart-like growth that crusts and occasionally bleeds

- a persistent, scaly, red, irregular patch that sometimes crusts or bleeds

- an open sore that bleeds and crusts and persists for weeks

- a rapidly developing elevated growth with a central depression that occasionally bleeds

♦ HUMAN PAPILLOMAVIRUS (HPV) AND DISEASE

There are more than 100 different types of HPV, most of which are harmless. Many people who have HPV show no symptoms. Some forms of HPV, however, can change normal epithelial cells into cancer cells. Cervical cancer is known to be caused by certain types of HPV. Other types of HPV have been linked to mouth and throat cancers and SCC of the skin. Research has shown that infection with the HPV may cause Bowen's disease in the genital area. Also, people with the rare inherited condition **epidermodysplasia verruciformis** may have an increased chance of getting skin cancer. This is an "autosomal recessive" disease, which begins in childhood. Affected individuals develop red papules that spread over the body as gray or yellow scales. The disease is associated with an impaired immune system. Of the 15 HPVs associated with this disease, four are thought to cause skin cancer.

HPV can also cause warts that can grow anywhere on the body. Skin warts are noncancerous growths that are very common. They appear as small,

DIAGNOSIS AND TREATMENT

Any abnormal skin growth should be referred promptly to a dermatologist for examination. If the diagnosis suggests an AK, early treatment will prevent it from developing into SCC. If the growth is AK or SCC *in situ*, the treatments are pretty much the same as for treating BCCs. The chance that a primary cutaneous SCC will recur is 8 percent. Early detection and treatment of SCC is crucial for a good outcome. Cryosurgery is the most widely used treatment for individual AKs, while simple excision is

white, beige, or brown skin growths almost anywhere on the body. Some cause small, painless, rough-surfaced warts found on the fingers and face, while others cause larger, more painful, and flatter warts that grow on the soles of the feet. In addition to skin warts, some HPVs can cause genital warts and HPVs are the most common cause of sexually transmitted infection in the world. There are thought to be 20 million people infected with HPV in the United States. Although skin warts and genital warts are treatable, they are not curable since the treatments do not get rid of the virus, only its symptoms.

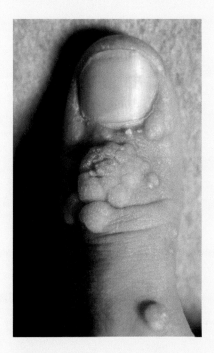

Figure 5.2 Warts are commonly found in children. (*Science VU/Visuals Unlimited*)

most common for treating SCCs *in situ*. **Immunotherapy** uses a topical cream, **imiquimod**, as a treatment for AK and Bowen's disease. Imiquimod causes cells to produce **interferon**, a natural chemical that attacks cancerous and precancerous cells and kills them. It is also used to treat warts. Laser surgery removes AKs from the face and scalp and actinic chelitis from the lips. This procedure is performed when topical treatments fail. Curettage and electrodessication are common procedures for treating AKs and SCCs: For AKs, only one procedure is required, while for SCCs, the procedure is repeated a number of times to ensure removal of all tumor cells. Radiation therapy using X-ray beams is used to destroy the tumor directly. Destruction usually requires several treatments a week for a few weeks. This is ideal for tumors that are hard to manage surgically and for elderly patients who are in poor health. Mohs micrographic surgery is often used to treat SCC *in situ* for the same reasons as for treating BCC. It also has the highest cure rate, causes the least amount of destruction to healthy tissue, and is carried out for recurrent tumors, and tumors in hard-to-treat places such as the head, neck, hands, and feet. Photodynamic Therapy (PDT) is used when SCCs appear on the face and scalp.

FROM SCC *IN SITU* TO METASTATIC SCC (MSCC)

In the general population, the rate of metastasis for a primary cutaneous SCC is 2 percent. For organ transplant recipients taking immunosuppressive drugs, the conversion to MSCC is approximately 10 percent. Also, in children who develop SCC *in situ*, 13 percent of these tumors will become metastatic, with an even higher risk if the original SCC developed on the lip or ear.

A "high-risk" SCC is defined as a tumor that is likely to metastasize to nearby lymph nodes based on unfavorable primary lesion features such as:

♦ tumors that have not been excised properly

♦ the size of the primary tumor—SCCs that recur locally and are more than 2 cm in diameter metastasize at a rate of 25 percent

♦ the tumor depth—there is a higher chance of metastasis if the tumor is more than 5 mm and has spread to the subcutaneous fat, muscle, or bone layers

- the "differentiated" state of the tumor; in general, cancers that resemble a more primitive (early) stage of the original cell type are more aggressive than cancers that appear more differentiated (i.e., more similar to the normal specialized cell type)

- SCCs arising in injured or chronically diseased skin are associated with a 40 percent increased risk of metastasis; also, the immunosuppression status of a person can play a huge part in determining the level of SCC risk

EPITHELIAL TO MESENCHYMAL TRANSITION

It is not clear what determines whether or not a SCC will metastasize. What is known is that the malignant conversion from SCC *in situ* to metastatic SCC requires a cell type conversion from the squamous cell (cuboidal) type to a more spindle-shaped, fibroblast-like cell type. This kind of malignant transformation is called epithelial to mesenchymal (connective tissue–like) transition (EMT). This process is common to many epithelial cancers (such as breast cancer), making them more aggressive. It occurs as a result of increasing genetic instability (more gene mutations) in the tumor, which promotes the cell changes to give rise to a more aggressive cancer.

TREATMENT OF MSCC

The long-term **prognosis** for SCC metastases is extremely poor. If the disease is found in the regional lymph nodes, the 10-year survival rate is less than 20 percent. In other words, fewer than 1 in 5 patients with regional lymph node SCC metastases survive past 10 years. If distant metastasis (when cancer has spread from the original tumor to distant organs or distant lymph nodes) is found, the 10-year survival rate is less than 10 percent. For SCC, 85 percent of metastases go the regional lymph nodes only, and approximately 15 percent of metastases involve distant sites, including the lungs, liver, brain, skin, and bone. "Staging" of the MSCC will determine which of the following courses of treatment should be given, and it is vital for patients to be monitored regularly over several years after initial treatment to make sure that the cancer does not recur.

SCC STAGING

The "Tumor-Node-Metastasis" or TNM classification system, as set out by American Joint Committee on Cancer, is used for staging SCC, as well as BCC.

TABLE 5.1 TUMOR-NODE-METASTASIS CLASSIFICATION SYSTEM		
CANCER SITE	CODE	DESCRIPTION
Primary tumor (T)	TX	Primary tumor cannot be assessed
	T0	No evidence of primary tumor
	Tis	Carcinoma in situ
	T1	Tumor ≤2 cm in greatest dimension
	T2	Tumor >2 cm but ≤5 cm
	T3	Tumor >5 cm
	T4	Tumor invades deeper structures (e.g., cartilage, skeletal muscle, or bone)
Regional lymph nodes (N)	NX	Regional lymph nodes cannot be assessed
	N0	No regional lymph node metastasis
	N1	Regional lymph node metastasis
Distant metastasis (M)	MX	Distant metastasis cannot be assessed
	M0	No distant metastasis
	M1	Distant metastasis

Further groupings of the above classifications are done by "stage":

TABLE 5.1 CANCER STAGING	
CATEGORY	STAGE
Stage 0	Tis, N0, M0
Stage I	T1, N0, M0
Stage II	T2, N0, M0; T3, N0, M0
Stage III	T4, N0, M0
Stage IV	Any T, N1, M0 Any T, any N, M1

Surgery is done when SCC is found in nodal metastases and around the nerves (i.e. Stage II–IV cancer), while radiotherapy is the primary treatment option in treating Stage III and IV SCC when tumors are inoperable. "Adjuvant" radiotherapy is often done in combination with surgery for metastatic or high-risk cutaneous SCC. **Adjuvant therapy** describes secondary treatments that increase the chances of curing a cancer. Chemotherapy with the most active chemotherapeutic agents—cisplatin, carboplatin, paclitaxel, docetaxel, 5-flurouracil, and methotrexate—is being used to treat metastatic cancers (i.e. Stage IV cancer). For treating advanced SCC, chemoradiotherapy, which combines standard chemotherapy and radiotherapy treatments, may be more beneficial. Finally, for organ transplant recipients, reduction of immunosuppressive drugs may be useful to prevent SCC development at all cancer stages, as long as it does not cause rejection of the transplanted organ.

FUTURE DIRECTIONS FOR TREATING METASTATIC SCC

Current treatments for nonmetastatic SCC are very effective, but once the SCC has metastasized, most treatments are ineffective. Chemotherapy is rarely done to treat the advanced cancer since it is rarely effective, but it is given to the patient to improve their quality of life (i.e. for palliative care). A potential new chemotherapy is rapamycin, an immunosuppressant with potent anticancer effects. Recent data suggest that it may decrease the risk of developing skin cancer and could perhaps be used instead of other immunosuppressant agents that are known to elevate skin cancer risks. Other future therapies for metastatic SCC are likely to include combinations of chemotherapy and radiation therapy.

SUMMARY

SCCs make up about 15 to 20 percent of all skin cancers. It is an epithelial cancer that develops from squamous cells in the spinous layer of the epidermis. The main risk factor for developing SCC is continuous exposure to UVR in sunlight. Caucasians and immunosuppressed people such as organ transplant patients who have to take immunosuppressive drugs, have a significantly higher chance of developing SCC than the rest of the human population. Although SCCs are very common, only a small proportion of these actually metastasize and cause death. SCC that has metastasized is very difficult to treat. Therefore, if detected and treated early, there is a good chance to recover fully from this cancer.

6

MELANOMA

KEY POINTS

♦ Melanoma is the deadliest skin cancer. More than 85 percent of skin cancer deaths are due to melanoma, although it makes up less than 5 percent of skin cancers.

♦ Melanomas arise from moles, which are clusters of melanin-containing melanocytes. Excessive sunburn during childhood is linked to developing melanoma.

♦ Early stage melanoma (Stage I melanoma) has a 100 percent survival rate.

♦ Advanced stage melanoma (Stage IV melanoma) has a 9 to 15 percent survival rate.

Melanoma is a disease that dates back to back to ancient times. The great Greek physician Hippocrates (born around 460 B.C.) who wrote the

Hippocratic Oath—the oath of ethical professional behavior that all new physicians must swear to when they start to practice medicine—was the first to be credited with reporting this disease, which he described as the "fatal black tumors with metastases." Evidence for the existence of melanoma in ancient times also comes from the discovery of melanoma tumors in the skin of Peruvian mummies that date to the fourth century B.C. The disease, however, was only named and described in detail in 1806, when the French physician René Laennec at the Le Faculté de Mediciné in Paris called it "la melanose."

Today, it is commonplace to hear about melanoma since many famous people have inadvertently drawn media attention to it. In 1998 at age 32, Troy Aikman, a quarterback who won three Super Bowls with the Dallas Cowboys, discovered a dime-shaped mole on his left shoulder blade that turned out to be melanoma. Luckily for him, his cancer was treatable and was removed promptly; he is living a melanoma-free life as a television sports commentator.

Another well-publicized melanoma survivor is John McCain, a Republican senator from Arizona. In 1993, McCain developed his first melanoma, which was successfully treated with no apparent further complications. In 2000, during his first presidential campaign, he underwent a routine check-up for skin cancer and it was discovered that he had two suspicious-looking moles on his arm and temple. These "moles" turned out to be melanoma, so McCain underwent immediate treatment, which involved a 5½-hour operation to remove the two melanomas and lymph nodes in his head and neck (to see whether the cancer had spread). His treatment was successful and although he has developed other melanomas since 2000, in 2007 he was melanoma-free and again campaigning for the U.S. presidency. During his childhood years and during the time spent as a prisoner-of-war during the Vietnam War, he sustained many blistering sunburns which undoubtedly significantly increased his chances of developing melanoma and other skin cancers. McCain is one of the fortunate survivors of melanoma, since this type of skin cancer kills one in six people who develop the disease.

The legendary Jamaican reggae singer-songwriter Bob Marley was not so fortunate and died of metastatic melanoma when he was only 36. In 1977, Marley visited a physician to have a wound on his left big toe checked out. It turned out to be a melanoma, and he was advised to have the toe amputated to prevent the cancer from spreading. He declined because of his Rastafarian beliefs (Rastafarianism is a religion and philosophy that accepts a former emperor of Ethiopia, Haile Selassie I, as a deity or godlike figure). In September 1980, Marley collapsed while jogging in Central Park in New York. Tests showed that his melanoma had metastasized to his brain, lungs, and stomach. He died eight months later in May 1981.

Melanoma is the deadliest form of skin cancer and makes up about 4 to 5 percent of all skin cancers. Almost all skin cancer deaths are due to melanoma, with an estimated 8,000 Americans dying from it every year. Although melanoma is relatively rare, it is one of the most common invasive cancers. While this cancer affects people of all ages with the risk increasing with age, it is one of the few cancers to affect young people, and is the third most common cancer among people who are 15 to 39 years old. For 2007, the National Cancer Institute (NCI) predicts that there will be approximately 60,000 new cases of melanoma in the United States, and approximately 8,110 of these will be fatal. This is an increase from previous years. Men are more likely to develop melanoma than women, and the lifetime risk of being diagnosed with melanoma is 1.77 percent for men and 1.25 percent for women.

MELANOMA ARISES FROM THE MELANOCYTES

Melanoma is a cancer of the pigment cells, the melanocytes, that produce the pigment melanin that is responsible for skin color and the tanning effect. Since this skin cancer does not develop from epithelial keratinocyte cells in the epidermis, melanoma can behave very differently from BCC and SCC. As with other skin cancers, however, the main cause of melanoma in four out of five cases is overexposure to ultraviolet radiation in sunlight, and this disease mainly affects fair-skinned Caucasian populations. The genetic damage caused by UVR is cumulative—that is, continuous chronic exposure to UVB (i.e., severe sunburns) from early childhood results in the accumulation of many damaging genetic mutations that eventually lead to melanoma. The UV exposure pattern for developing melanoma is similar to that for developing BCC. That is, intense intermittent UV exposure resulting in sunburn, rather than continuous UV exposure (as for SCC), especially in childhood, most likely causes melanoma to develop.

MOLES AND MELANOMA

In general, melanoma arises from small pigmented moles, or nevi, on the skin (Figure 6.1). Moles arise due to the clumping together of melanocytes in the skin. Most do not form tumors and are therefore referred to as "benign nevi." Occasionally, some of these may acquire damaging genetic mutations (caused by exposure to UVR, for example) and become abnormal, developing into a primary melanoma tumor. Most melanomas start as slow growing tumors that spread horizontally only in the epidermis and extend upwards. This is known as "pagetoid spread" and melanomas that grow like this are in the **radial growth phase** (**RGP**). These tumors are *in situ* and do not invade the dermis,

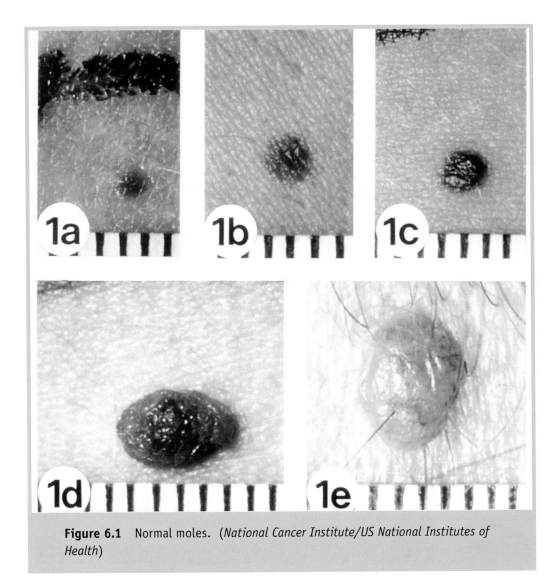

Figure 6.1   Normal moles.   (*National Cancer Institute/US National Institutes of Health*)

and are unlikely to metastasize. If the melanoma progresses, however, it undergoes a **vertical growth phase** (**VGP**) and invades the dermis and deeper tissues. When the melanoma does this, there is a good chance that it can metastasize. If not treated early, this tumor may develop into metastatic melanoma that will eventually spread throughout the body.

NONCUTANEOUS MELANOMA

Melanoma can develop in nonskin areas of the body that contain pigment cells, such as the eyes, digestive tract, and lymph nodes. These melanomas are extremely rare compared to cutaneous melanoma. Ocular melanoma (melanoma of the eye) sometimes behaves differently from melanoma of the skin and other parts of the body. Melanoma of the mouth—the most common form of melanoma in Japanese people—is usually found when the tumor is "thick" and more advanced since it is hidden in the mouth and escapes early detection.

♦ THE MOLE AS A BEAUTY MARK

The concept of the mole as a sign of beauty probably dates to Renaissance times (fourteenth through sixteenth centuries), and was particularly popular with French women in the eighteenth century, when natural or artificial moles on the face were considered feminine and attractive. In the twentieth century, the mole again gained prominence among the fashionable when the movie star Marilyn Monroe sported a facial mole just above her lip, along her dimple line. Although her mole was thought to be real, these days many celebrities use make-up to "draw in" facial moles to copy the "Marilyn Monroe beauty spot" look. In general, moles are considered most attractive if they are found on the face within an inch or so of the upper lip or around the eyes. Moles found elsewhere on the body are not considered attractive.

RISK FACTORS FOR MELANOMA

The exact causes of cutaneous melanoma are unknown, but the main risk factors for developing this disease are well established. Many of them overlap extensively with factors that cause nonmelanoma skin cancer and include: a) overexposure to UV radiation, either natural or artificial sources; b) race—Caucasians are most susceptible to developing melanoma; c) having many moles; d) family history of melanoma—10 percent of affected patients have an affected relative; e) personal history of melanoma or other skin cancers; f) a weakened immune system due to illness; and g) history of severe blistering sunburns from childhood.

GENETICS OF MELANOMA

Familial Melanoma/Dysplastic Nevus Syndrome

Familial melanoma (FM), or dysplastic nevus syndrome (DNS), is an inherited disease in which individuals have a high risk of developing melanoma. These people make up 5 to 10 percent of patients diagnosed with melanoma, and they often have at least one family member who also has melanoma. These people develop atypical (abnormal) nevi that show histological features of a benign but possibly precancerous condition (dysplasia). These dysplastic nevi are good indicators of melanoma risk. FM/DNS individuals with dysplastic nevi have a lifetime risk of developing melanoma that approaches 100 percent.

FM/DNS has been linked to a gene on chromosome 9, called *p16* (also known as *CDKN2A*, *CDKN2*, *MTS1*, and *INK4A*). As an important regulator of cell division, p16 protein acts as a brake on cell cycle progression. It inhibits proteins called cyclin dependent kinases (CDK4 and CDK6), which promote cell proliferation. If p16 is not working properly in a melanocyte, the latter will proliferate uncontrollably.

Eventually, the proliferations are seen collectively as a new or larger mole, which can develop into melanoma. Laboratory experiments investigating the loss of p16 function suggests that p16 may prevent moles from becoming malignant.

The *BRAF* Gene and Melanoma

In 2002, researchers in Great Britain identified the gene *BRAF* (pronounced "B-raf") as a causal factor of melanoma. *BRAF* is a gene that makes a protein that promotes cell growth. It is mutated in about 60 to 70 percent of most melanomas. The mutation makes the BRAF protein active all the time so that it no longer responds to signals that should turn it off. Therefore, melanocytes with the *BRAF* mutation can multiply unchecked and develop into melanoma.

DETECTION AND DIAGNOSIS

Everyone has normal moles, which are generally noncancerous. They can be present at birth or they can appear later, in small or large numbers. A normal mole is often an evenly colored brown, tan, or black spot on the skin, which can appear either flat or raised, round or oval, and is usually less than 0.25 inch (0.6 cm) in diameter (Figure 6.1). Once a mole has developed, it will usually stay the same size, shape, and color for many years, or may fade away (for unknown reasons) in older people.

Melanoma may develop on any skin surface. For men, the most common areas are the trunk and, to a lesser extent, the head and neck. For women, the most common area is the lower legs, followed by the trunk. Melanoma is rare in dark-skinned individuals, but these people may develop the disease under fingernails or toenails, or on the palms or soles of the feet, where the skin is lighter. Many people will

---

◆ DOGS THAT DETECT MELANOMA

In 1989, the British journal *Lancet* suggested that dogs may be able to sniff out cancer. The journal describes a woman whose her dog had "expressed exceptional interest" (by excessive sniffing) in a skin lesion on her leg. This skin lesion turned out to be malignant melanoma. Since this report was published, many anecdotal stories of dogs detecting skin cancer and internal cancers such as those of the breast and lung have been reported. The idea that dogs can smell cancer is not unreasonable, since tumors produce specific volatile organic compounds (such as the alkanes, ethane and pentane) that are released through breath and sweat. These compounds may have distinctive odors, which collectively form a signature smell of cancer that may be detected by dogs, since they have exceptional olfactory ability.

---

visit a dermatologist when they notice a change in an existing mole. This change may be in its shape, size, and/or color. An excision biopsy is carried out to check that the mole is melanoma (a shave biopsy is not recommended if the tumor looks like a melanoma since this biopsy may not be sufficient to find out how deeply the cancer has penetrated into the skin tissues). Better education about skin cancer has prompted people to perform regular self-examinations of their skin. New ways to detect malignant melanoma are also being explored.

HOW TO DETECT A POTENTIAL MELANOMA

The general things to consider when looking for possible melanomas are outlined with the ABCD method:

Asymmetry: When the shape of one half of the mole does not match the other.

Border: When the edges of the mole are ragged, notched, blurred, or irregular in outline, or the pigment may have spread into the surrounding skin.

Color: When moles have an uneven color, with shades of black, brown, tan, or areas of white, gray, red, pink, or blue. On occasion, melanoma can be the same color as the rest of the skin.

Diameter: Melanomas are usually larger than the eraser of a pencil (6 millimeters in diameter), but smaller moles that have other characteristics as outlined in the ABCD method, or itch and/or bleed should be examined by a dermatologist.

The ABCD method can help people identify suspicious growths since melanomas can take various appearances. The only way to definitively diagnose melanoma is to have a biopsy performed by a doctor.

METASTATIC OR NONMETASTATIC?

Once a growth has been confirmed as melanoma, the doctor needs to establish whether the tumor is a melanoma *in situ* or whether it has spread. The staging of the cancer at diagnosis is critical in determining the kind of treatment to be administered. Cutaneous melanoma can be divided into subcategories based on its anatomical location and its pattern of growth. Melanoma staging is generally done for all confirmed melanomas and is carried out by looking to see how deep into the skin the tumor has developed and whether the tumor has spread to regional lymph nodes or distant sites. Generally, melanoma can be cured if it is diagnosed and treated when the tumor is thin and has not invaded deeply. When a melanoma is thick and deep in the skin, the disease has often spread to the lymph nodes and other parts of the body. There are,

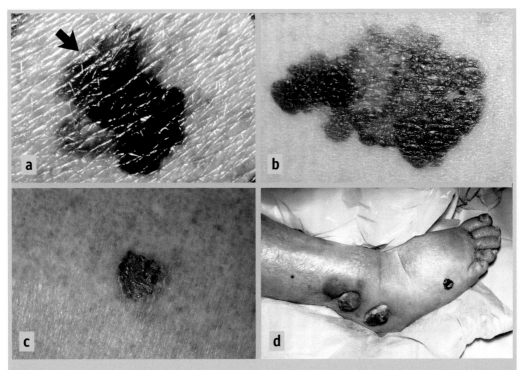

Figure 6.2 Various forms of Melanoma. Melanomas *in situ* are often pigmented and have an irregular border (a–c). Malignant melanoma (d). (*National Cancer Institute/US National Institutes of Health; Dr. Ken Greer/Visuals Unlimited; Mediscan/Visuals Unlimited*)

however, problems with staging melanoma using thickness since many thin melanomas have been found to have spread and only 40 percent of the thicker type generally spread. In a finding published in 2004 in the *British Journal of Cancer*, researchers in Great Britain suggested a new method to determine whether melanoma is likely to metastasize. This method works by measuring the density of the lymph vessels around melanomas: The denser they are, the greater the chance that the melanoma is metastatic.

Other histological aspects determine the prognosis, such as **mitotic index** (the ratio of the number of cells undergoing **mitosis** compared to the number of cells not undergoing mitosis), presence of tumor-infiltrating lymphocytes, the number of regional lymph nodes involved, and ulceration or bleeding at the primary tumor site. Melanoma can spread through the lymphatic system and/or through the bloodstream to distant sites. Any organ may be invaded by melanoma metastases, but the lungs and the liver are the common sites. To see where the cancer has spread, a dye can be injected into the primary tumor site. Following where the dye goes will give some indication of the amount and pattern of the cancer's spread.

Melanoma Staging

There are many staging systems for melanoma, which can cause confusion even among professionals who diagnose the cancer. Therefore, it is generally advisable to get a second opinion on a melanoma staging to prevent misdiagnosis. For initial staging, there is the Clark's Classification (Level of Invasion) outlined in Table 6.1 on the next page.

More extensive staging, such as the TNM- and the Clinical staging systems, which are similar to those described in Chapter 5 but with more sub-classifications. Another classification system is Breslow depth staging, which refer to the microscopic depth of tumor invasion. All these staging systems are outlined on the Web site of the National Cancer Institute of the United States.

TREATMENTS FOR MELANOMA *IN SITU*

Up to 85 percent of all melanoma patients are diagnosed with early stage (Stage 0) disease, which is the least aggressive and most treatable type. Indeed, there is a 100 percent survival rate when the melanoma is treated

TABLE 6.1 CLARK'S CLASSIFICATION (LEVEL OF INVASION)	
LEVEL	DESCRIPTION
0	The melanoma cells are found only in the epidermis and have not invaded deeper tissues. It is a melanoma *in situ*.
I	The tumor is no more than 1 millimeter thick and the epidermis may appear ulcerated ("scraped"), or the tumor is between 1 and 2 millimeters with no ulceration. The cancer has not spread to the nearby lymph nodes.
II	The tumor is between 1 and 2 millimeters thick with ulceration, or the tumor is more than 2 millimeters thick with no ulceration. There is invasion into the dermis but the cancer has not spread to the nearby lymph nodes.
III	The tumor has spread to tissues next to the original tumor but not to any lymph nodes, or the melanoma cells have spread to one or more nearby lymph nodes.
IV	The melanoma cells have spread to the lymph nodes and to other organs, or to skin areas far from the original tumor.

at this stage. Treatments for primary melanomas are similar to those described for BCC and SCC. The most common and successful way to treat early-stage melanoma is with surgery to remove the tumor. Generally, the disease does not progress further after surgical removal of the Stage 0 melanoma. For melanomas that are Stages I or II, the treatment is also surgical removal of the tumor, and 85 to 95 percent of patients survive beyond five years. For Stages II and III melanoma, the five-year survival rate is 40 to 85 percent and 25 to 60 percent, respectively. When the melanoma becomes a Stage II/III cancer, surgery to remove the tumor and the surrounding normal tissue is carried out. Sometimes the nearby lymph nodes are removed as a precaution. This procedure is known as lymph node dissection (lymphectomy). There are two types of lymph node dissection: therapeutic and elective. Therapeutic dissection involves surgical removal of the diseased lymph node, while elective dissection involves removal of the lymph nodes that have the potential to develop metastases but have not yet done so. This is a controversial treatment since it is unclear whether it actually prevents the spread of the disease. Chemotherapy is also sometimes used to kill the cancer cells, as is immunotherapy, which uses cytokines, a component of the body's own immune system, to fight the cancer. Early detection and treatment of melanoma is vital since melanoma metastasizes to remote body sites even when the tumor is relatively small and thin, and once it has metastasized, the cancer is characteristically unresponsive to treatment.

TREATMENTS FOR METASTATIC MELANOMA

For patients diagnosed with metastatic melanoma, the outlook is not very good—the average survival time is six to 10 months after diagnosis and the five-year survival rate is 9 to 15 percent. At this stage, melanoma is difficult to control, since it is highly aggressive and resists conventional therapies. To check whether the nearby lymph nodes contain cancer cells, they are either removed, or some tissue or fluid is collected from the nodes and analyzed. If the lymph nodes contain metastases, several treatments may be used. It is based on the theory that like other metastatic cancers, melanomas often spread sequentially from the primary melanoma tumor to the nearby lymph nodes and then to more distant parts of the body.

Metastatic melanoma is highly resistant to chemotherapy. At present, the only drugs with some effect against this disease are dacarbazine

(DTIC) and the nitrosoureas, carmustine (BCNU) and lomustine. The response rate is only about 10 to 20 percent and the response is short-lived, although a small number of patients have completely responded to treatment. Therefore more effective therapies are needed to combat this aggressive disease.

Existing cancer therapies that utilize the body's own immune system (immunotherapy) are being tested in people with advanced cases of melanoma. These include the use of interferon alpha (IFN-α), which is also being used to treat BCC and SCC, and **interleukin-2 (IL-2)**, which stimulates the growth and activity of immune cells that can destroy cancer cells. Therapies are also being developed using therapeutic melanoma **vaccines** designed to help the body's immune system to recognize and attack melanoma cancer cells without harming normal cells. Research has shown that many cancers, including melanoma, express protein markers (**antigens**) that are not present in normal cells and that can be recognized as "foreign" by the body's immune system, which targets the cancer for destruction.

POST-TREATMENT FOR METASTATIC MELANOMA

The five-year survival rates for regional and distant stage metastatic melanomas are 64 percent and 16 percent, respectively (compared to 98 percent for localized melanoma). Once the metastatic cancer is treated, the patient is carefully monitored to see whether he or she will relapse. The risk of relapse from a metastatic melanoma decreases substantially after a long time has passed (at least five years), though late relapses are not uncommon. Patients who are younger and female, and who have melanomas on the extremities, generally have a good prognosis of the initial melanoma not recurring, compared to patients that are older and male.

SUMMARY

Melanoma is the deadliest skin cancer and is the main cause of skin-cancer-related deaths. When treated early, melanoma can generally be cured. For those melanomas that advance and develop into metastatic melanoma, however, the outcome is not good, since this disease is highly resistant to current therapies. Clinical trials of several new drugs for metastatic melanoma are being conducted, but it will be years before we know whether they will be able to cure or even just manage this cancer. Therefore, the best way to manage this disease is to promote preventive measures such as avoiding excessive exposure to the sun's ultraviolet rays and by avoiding artificial tanning beds. Indeed, prevention of melanoma is probably the best way to avoid the disease.

7

OTHER SKIN CANCERS AND RELATED CONDITIONS

KEY POINTS

- Cells in the skin other than epidermal cells and melanocytes can develop into cancer.

- These cancers are generally rare and can be benign or malignant and metastatic.

- There are many noncancer conditions that increase the chances of developing skin cancer.

In 2006 a documentary, *The Girl Who Lives In The Dark*, was made about a nine-year-old girl from China, Wao Lao Yang. She has the rare genetic disorder xeroderma pigmentosum (XP), which prevents her skin from repairing itself after exposure to ultraviolet radiation. The documentary tells how she had "weeping sores" on her face, which produced an unpleasant smell caused by bacteria surrounding the skin tumors. It was so bad that she could not go outdoors, attend school, or even watch television. Her village doctor tried to treat her with natural herbs, which, unsurprisingly, had no effect, so she was sent to Shanghai and then to the world-famous Great Ormond Street Children's Hospital in London for treatment. There, she underwent advanced surgeries and was fitted with a "sunsuit" made by NASA (National Aeronautics and Space Administration) scientists that completely blocked ultraviolet radiation. When she went home to China, her home and school were fitted with UV-filtered windows so she could live a relatively "normal" life with the disease. Life, however, will never be normal since the disease has left her severely disfigured and Wao Lao will never be able to enjoy the outdoors in the same way most people can.

XP is one of a number of diseases that are associated with developing many skin cancers. These skin-cancer associated conditions are not common but can be very severe. In addition, there are generally rare types of skin cancer that develop from cells other than keratinocytes and melanocytes. Some of these are benign cancers, like most BCCs and SCCs, while others are highly malignant, like metastatic melanoma. We will outline some examples of these rare skin-associated cancers and diseases in this chapter. Also included in this chapter is a basosquamous carcinoma, which does not exclusively fit the criteria of being a BCC or an SCC, and has an ambigious classification.

BASOSQUAMOUS CARCINOMA (BSC)

This is a metastatic cancer that is still not well defined. It is a very rare skin cancer that has characteristics of BCCs and SCCs and has significant potential to metastasize. BSC is most commonly found in the head and neck region, and less commonly in the trunk and limbs. The incidence of BSC is not well defined. It has been suggested that BSCs make up approximately 2 percent of all skin carcinomas and that they have a greater potential to metastasize compared to BCCs and possibly even SCCs. More men are thought to develop this type of cancer than women, and the average age of onset is about 70 years old.

Initially, scientists and clinicians were not sure whether BSC was a distinct form of cancer. Many people thought that BSC was the collision of separate primary BCC and SCC lesions that were located close together, or a BCC with the ability to form keratin, which is commonly seen for a more differentiated SCC. These "collision tumors" and "keratinizing BCC" do, in fact, exist. Since BSC's classification is ambiguous, the most appropriate treatment for it remains to be established. The current treatment is based on therapies for both BCC and SCC. Generally, a wide local excision of the tumor and an evaluation for metastasis to lymph nodes and distant sites are done. This is followed by a careful check-up to look for recurrence and metastasis. Prevention of BSC recurrence is important and can be predicted to some degree by looking at the tumor margins (the region where the tumor contacts the normal tissue) of the removed tumor. If the margins are positive for tumor cells, the tumor recurrence is likely. Also lymphatic invasion and perineural invasion (when tumor cells surround the nerves) by tumor cells is an indication that the cancer is likely to recur. Furthermore, if the patient is male and the tumor size greater than 2 cm, there is a likelihood of the cancer recurring. As with other potentially recurring cancers, adjuvant therapy is given. This is therapy given after the primary treatment to increase the chances of a cure. It is given in the form of topical fluorouracil (5-FU) and radiation therapy, based on the fact that BSC is similar to BCC and SCC.

SKIN-ASSOCIATED CANCERS

There are cells in the skin other than the keratinocytes and the melanocytes that may have the potential to develop into cancer. These include cells of the sweat gland, sebaceous gland, fat layer, and of the nerves.

Cancers of the sweat gland are generally very rare and can be either benign or metastatic. Benign sweat gland cancers include adenoma, an epithelial sweat gland cancer, and syringoma, which develops from well-differentiated ductal elements in the sweat gland. Syringoma are relatively common—affecting mainly women—and usually form small, yellow or red-brown, firm clusters of papules on the eyelid. People with Down's syndrome (a mental retardation syndrome caused by having an extra chromosome) have a higher rate of this cancer. Sweat gland cancers that have the potential to metastasize include porocarcinoma, syringoid carcinoma, ductal carcinoma, adenoid cystic carcinoma, and mucinous carcinoma. Porocarcinoma is rare and develops on the lower extremities of older people. It may be a verrucous (wart-like) plaque or it may be ulcerated. Syringoid carcinoma resembles primary cancers of the lung, salivary gland, and breast, while ductal carcinoma has tubular growths with solid masses of tumor "nests." Adenoid cystic carcinoma are rare and appears as dermal basaloid growths, while mucinous carcinoma show sweat gland differentiation and produce mucin, which are large, secreted proteins. Nonmetastatic tumors can be removed by wide local excision. For syringoma, a suggested treatment is to use a hair removal electric needle, which emits short bursts of low voltage electricity to remove the tumor.

SEBACEOUS GLAND CARCINOMA

Sebaceous gland carcinoma (SGC) is a very rare type of skin cancer of the sebaceous gland. The incidence of this cancer is 3.2 percent among malignant tumors and it is generally found in women in their 70s. It is a highly aggressive, metastatic cancer (the death rate is 22 percent) that can occur in any skin that has sebaceous glands, such as the follicular epidermis. Three-quarters of these cancers appear in the eye region, however, with the most common site being the upper eyelid. Metastasis occurs in 14 to 25 percent of all SGC tumors, first to the nearby lymph nodes and then to distant sites such as the liver, bones, and brain. The cause of SGC is not fully understood. Usually, the affected person also has another type of cancer elsewhere in the body. SGC is associated with noncancerous lumps of the sebaceous glands, exposure to radiation, such as previous radiotherapy or (less likely) repeated X rays, and Muir-Torré syndrome, a rare genetic disease. The treatments for this cancer are similar to those described for metastatic cancers: Surgical excision is normally carried out, followed by lymph node evaluation to check for metastasis.

LIPOMA

Lipoma is a benign fatty skin tumor that may grow quickly at first and then remain unchanged for years. Strictly speaking, it is a subcutaneous "soft-tissue" tumor. Lipomas are the most common subcutaneous soft-tissue tumors, affecting about 1 in 1,000 people in the United States each year. Lipoma is commonly found in adults from 40 to 60 years of age but can also be found in children. They are generally slow-growing nodules with a firm, rubbery consistency. These tumors commonly appear on the trunk, neck, and shoulders, and can develop after mild physical injury. Tumors are not generally removed unless they cause compression and/or physical disfigurement. When they are removed, the tumors are generally cut out or "squeezed" out through a small incision. Alternatively, they can be removed by liposuction (the removal of excess body fat by suction with specialized surgical equipment).

MERKEL CELL CARCINOMA

Merkel cell carcinoma (MCC) is a rare aggressive, neuroendocrine (has characteristics of both neural and endocrine cells) cancer of the skin. There are approximately 1,200 new cases in the United States every year. MCC is usually found on or just beneath the skin and in hair follicles, and on the sun-exposed areas of the head, neck, arms, and legs. Caucasian people between ages 60 and 80 years generally develop this cancer, although some cases have been reported in Japanese people. Very few cases of this cancer have been reported in black people. Tumors usually appear as firm, painless, shiny lumps of skin, which can be red, pink, or blue, varying in size from 0.25 inches (0.64 centimeters) to more than 2 inches (5.08 centimeters). This cancer can be difficult to diagnose because it resembles other cancers, especially some cancers of the lung, which have neuroendocrine features. MCC has the tendency to metastasize to nearby lymph nodes and to other areas, including the liver, bones, lungs, and brain. Treatment depends on the stage of the disease, and the patient's age and overall physical condition. Although treatment may shrink the tumor, it will not cure the patient of this cancer. Therefore, it is common for MCC to recur.

KAPOSI'S SARCOMA

Kaposi's **sarcoma** (KS) was named after Moritz Kaposi, a Hungarian physician and dermatologist at the University of Vienna, Austria, who first described it in 1872. It is a soft connective-tissue cancer that causes cutaneous tumors on the extremities or tumors in the mucous membranes of the mouth, nose, and anus. Tumors appear as raised blotches or as purple, brown, or red nodules. The disease is not usually life-threatening or disabling, but it may be very disfiguring and painful due to swelling. KS only becomes life-threatening when it affects the lungs, liver, or gastrointestinal tract, since it can cause bleeding in the abdomen or breathing difficulties if the tumors occur in the lungs.

There are a few different categories of KS. Classic Kaposi's sarcoma usually affects Jewish and Italian men of European descent between the ages of 50 and 70. Patients typically have one or more tumors on the limbs. Pressure from these growths can block lymph vessels, causing painful swelling. African (endemic) KS is commonly found in people living in equatorial Africa. It affects more men than women. It accounts for 9 percent of all the cancers seen among men in Uganda and is identical to classic KS except that it strikes at a much younger age. This form of KS causes **asymptomatic** skin lesions and does not spread to other parts of the body. More aggressive cases can occur, however, with some tumors penetrating from the skin to the underlying bone. Transplant-related (acquired) KS occurs in people who have had organ transplants. People whose immune systems have been suppressed are 150 to 200 times more likely to develop KS than the general population. KS in these patients mainly affects the skin. AIDS-related Kaposi's sarcoma affects people who are HIV-positive or have AIDS. The damage to the immune system caused by the virus (Figure 7.1) makes them more susceptible to developing KS.

CONDITIONS RELATED TO SKIN-CANCER

There are several diseases and medical conditions that can be directly associated with developing skin cancer. These conditions increase a

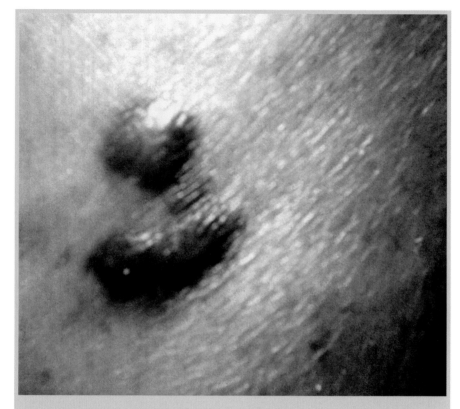

Figure 7.1   Kaposi's sarcoma on an AIDS patient.   (*CDC/Dr. Steve Kraus*)

person's susceptibility to developing greater numbers of skin cancers than the general population.

Xeroderma Pigmentosum

Xeroderma pigmentosum (XP) was first described in 1874 by Ferdinand Hebra and Moritz Kaposi (the same physician who described Kaposi's sarcoma) at the University of Vienna. They named the disease because it caused the skin to be dry and pigmented. XP is a rare, inherited,

◆ HIV AND AIDS

Acquired immunodeficiency syndrome (AIDS) was first reported in 1981. Since then, more than 900,000 cases of AIDS have been diagnosed in the United States. AIDS is caused by the human immunodeficiency virus (HIV), a blood-borne pathogen that destroys certain cells of the immune system, leaving the body unable to fight off infections. It is generally sexually transmitted, but people can also get it from contaminated hypodermic needles. The virus can also be transmitted from an infected mother to her unborn child.

A person infected with HIV does not necessarily have AIDS. Full-blown AIDS begins when the virus has caused serious damage to the immune system, leading to the development of many life-threatening infections and medical complications. As many as 950,000 Americans may be infected with HIV. It is a leading killer of African-American males between the ages of 25 and 44. AIDS patients are particularly prone to developing cancers such as Kaposi's sarcoma, cervical cancer, and cancers of the immune system.

autosomal recessive disease caused by a mutation in a gene that codes for an enzyme involved in repairing UVR-induced DNA damage. XP occurs equally in males and females and in all races. Affected individuals are normally diagnosed at age one or two, when a short sun exposure results in severe sunburn due to their extreme sensitivity to sunlight. Affected children have to be completely shielded from the sun, and are often referred to as "children of the night," since night is the only time that they can safely play outdoors without severely damaging their skin.

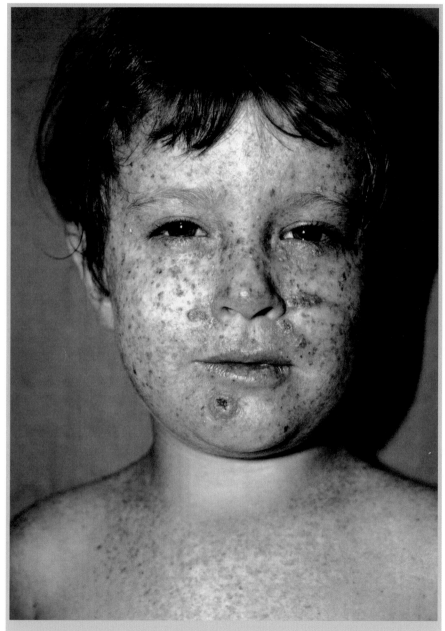

Figure 7.2   Xeroderma pigmentosum patient.   (*Dr. Ken Greer/Visuals Unlimited*)

In addition to the severe blistering that occurs with sun exposure, XP-affected individuals are very susceptible to developing skin cancer. The average age of onset is eight years old, compared to 50 to 60 years old for people without XP. Patients younger than 20 years of age have a thousandfold increase in the incidence of nonmelanoma skin cancer and melanoma. Many children with XP die from metastatic melanoma or metastatic SCC. In the United States, there is approximately one case of XP per 250,000 people.

Organ Failure

People with organ failure require a replacement organ to stay alive. It is now fairly commonplace to remove an organ from someone who has recently died, or from a living person donating an organ, and place it into another person to save his or her life. A huge problem with donated organs, however, is that there is a high risk that the recipient's body will "reject" it as a foreign object and send immune cells to destroy it. To prevent this, an organ from a blood relative is preferred over one from a nonblood-related donor, since the organ will be more genetically compatible with the recipient and is less likely to be rejected. If there is some level of incompatibility, however, immunosuppressive drugs must be taken to prevent organ rejection, and this comes with a high risk of developing skin cancer, such as SCC. As mentioned in Chapter 5, rapamycin, an immunosuppressant drug, has been shown in the laboratory to have anti-cancer properties. If further scientific studies show that it has effects against SCC, rapamycin could potentially be used as a standard treatment to prevent organ rejection without increasing the rate of skin cancer in organ transplant patients.

◆ DIFFERENT TYPES OF GRAFTS

An organ transplant is the replacement of a whole or partial organ from one body with one from another body (or from a donor site on the patient's own body) to replace the recipient's damaged or failing organ. Organ donors can be living or deceased. There are various types of transplants:

Autograft: This is when tissue from a person's own body is transplanted to another part of the body. The graft is usually taken from areas with surplus tissue (such as the buttocks) and/or from tissue that can regenerate. For example, the skin is a common tissue for autografts in cases of severe burns. Autografts sometimes involve removing the tissue and then treating it or the person before returning the graft to its original place.

Isograft: This type of graft involves transplanting organs or tissues from one person to a genetically identical other (such as an identical twin).

Allograft: This is a transplanted organ or tissue from a genetically nonidentical member of the same **species**. Most human tissue and organ transplants are allografts.

Xenograft: This is a transplant of organs or tissue from one species to another. These kinds of grafts have been successfully used in heart-valve transplants from pigs to humans. Heart transplants from baboons to humans have been tried and were unsuccessful.

Lymphoma

Lymphoma is a cancer of the lymphatic system, which is part of the immune system and consists of a network of thin vessels and nodes spread throughout the body. The lymphatic system is important for fighting off infections. Lymphoma develops when white blood cells called lymphocytes, which normally fight off infectious agents, mutate and turn into cancer. There are two types of cutaneous (skin) lymphomas: the more common T-cell lymphoma, which arises from the T-lymphocytes, and B-cell lymphoma, which develops from the B-lymphocytes.

Cutaneous T-cell lymphoma (CTCL), also known as mycosis fungoides, is a T-cell lymphoma that affects the skin. It makes up 65 percent of all skin lymphomas and is generally confined to the skin. The incidence of CTCL is estimated at 0.5 to 1 cases per 100,000 people. CTCL targets the skin, since it is attracted by a variety of antigens found there (these may be skin antigens, viruses, bacteria, or fungi) and is stimulated to divide. Left untreated, CTCL can remain in the skin for years, but it may eventually metastasize to the lymph nodes, blood, or internal organs. As with other cancers that may metastasize, early-stage CTCL is curable, while late-stage metastatic CTCL does not respond well to current treatments. The treatments available for CTCL include phototherapy, which uses UVB and UVA (however, this treatment is risky since UVA and UVB exposure increases the risk of other skin cancers); chemotherapy using **topical nitrogen mustard**, which can induce long-term remission and even cures; extracorporeal photochemotherapy (ECP), in which some of the patient's white blood cells are removed from the body, treated with UVA light, then returned to the patient's body; and electron-beam therapy, which is high-energy radiation that affects only the skin and does not penetrate to the internal organs. Complete cancer remission occurs in about 84 percent of CTCL individuals treated with this therapy, but the cancer often returns as a more advanced disease. In CTCL patients with advanced CTCL, chemotherapy is typically used only to alleviate pain.

SUMMARY

In our skin there are cells other than the epidermal keratinocyte cells and the melanocytes that can give rise to skin cancers. In general, they are not as common as BCC and SCC, or even melanoma, and these cancers can be either benign, or highly aggressive and metastatic. In addition to these skin cancers, there are medical conditions that are not cancers but may result in an increased rate of skin cancers. People with these conditions may need to take preventive measures to decrease their chances of getting skin cancer.

8

SKIN CANCER PREVENTION

KEY POINTS

♦ Skin cancer is by far the most preventable of all cancers.

♦ Skin cancer is mainly caused by excessive exposure to the sun's ultraviolet rays.

♦ Simple measures such as protective clothing, sunscreens, and sun avoidance in the afternoon can significantly decrease our chances of developing skin cancer.

♦ Prevention is best way to avoid getting skin cancer.

Skin cancer is the most preventable form of cancer. Despite this, approximately one million new cases of basal and squamous cell cancers and about 60,000 new cases of malignant melanoma were diagnosed in the United States in 2005, and about 8,000 deaths resulted from metastatic melanoma. A survey published in 2001 in the *American Journal of*

Preventive Medicine found that about 43 percent of Caucasian children under the age of 12 had at least one sunburn during the past year. If they continued to do so at the same rate throughout life, this would greatly increase their chances of getting skin cancer.

In general, most people do not take enough precautions to protect themselves from skin cancer. Therefore, we need better education about the hazards of ultraviolet radiation and on ways to protect ourselves since most skin cancers are caused by chronic sun exposure. For reasons outlined in Chapter 3, Australia has the highest rate of skin cancer in the world. In 1981, one of the most successful health campaigns in Australia's history was launched. The "Slip Slop Slap" campaign spread the message to schools and communities that sun protection prevents skin cancer. It educated young people to "Slip on a shirt, slop on sunscreen, and slap on a hat," and it was largely credited with curbing the dramatic increase in skin cancer that was seen about 20 years ago. As the Australian "Slip Slop Slap" campaign suggests, there are a number of straightforward approaches we can take to reduce overexposure to sunlight and avoid skin cancer.

AVOIDING INTENSE SUNLIGHT

It is important to perform outdoor activities on a regular basis, but it is also important to limit your exposure to intense sunlight. From 10:00 A.M. until 4:00 P.M., the sun's UV rays are at their most intense. Therefore, you should spend less time outside during these hours. A good way to tell when the sun's rays are at their strongest is to look at your shadow. If your shadow is shorter than you are, then the sun is too strong for lengthy exposure. The Environmental Protection Agency (EPA) and National Weather Service have Web sites on which you can find out how intense the UV rays are in your area.

Other factors, such as altitude, ambient temperature, pollution, wind, and medication can affect a person's sensitivity to sunlight. If a person's medication has the possibility to increase his or her sensitivity to sunlight, this will be indicated in the documentation that comes with the medication. People who take such medications need to take extra measures to protect themselves from intense sunlight. If sun avoidance is not possible, then other precautionary measures should be taken.

Protective Clothing

If going out in intense sunlight is unavoidable, you should wear clothing to cover as much skin as possible, such as long-sleeved shirts, long pants, or long skirts. Wearing dark colors provides more protection than light colors, since dark colors prevent more UV rays from reaching your skin, as do fabrics that are tightly woven and opaque (impenetrable to light). If you can see light through a fabric, then UVR can get through too. We are often told, however, to wear light-colored clothes in hot weather; this is because light-colored clothes keep us cooler, since they do not absorb as much heat as dark-colored clothes. Ideal sun-protective fabrics are lightweight and comfortable, and protect against exposure even when wet.

Hats with at least a 2- to 3-inch (5- to 7.6-cm) brim all around are good for protecting areas that are often exposed to the sun, such as the neck, ears, eyes, forehead, nose, and scalp. Although people commonly wear baseball caps in the sun, these caps only provide protection for the front and top of the head, not the back of the neck or the ears, where skin cancers often develop.

Eye protection is also important to reduce damage from intense UV radiation. Generally, wearing UV-absorbent sunglasses can help protect the eyes from sun damage, which may be associated with the

---

◆ THE UV INDEX

The UV index was devised by the Environmental Protection Agency and the National Weather Service to tell people the amount of UV radiation that is reaching the earth at noon. The index number ranges from 0 to 11+ ("+" meaning "greater than 11"). The higher the number, the greater the UVR exposure. For example, 11+ indicates that UVR exposure will be very high and skin protection is needed. The index is forecast daily for 58 cities in the United States and is based on locally predicted weather conditions. You can find out the UV index for your region by visiting the EPA's Web site (http://www.epa.gov/sunwise/uvindex.html).

---

development of ocular melanoma. It is important to buy sunglasses only if they have a label indicating that they have met safety standards. Not all sunglasses are equal in their ability to protect your eyes from UVR. Also, it is important to point out that darker glasses do not necessarily provide better protection, since the UV protection comes from a chemical that is applied to the lenses. The best shape of sunglasses is the large-framed "wraparound" sunglasses that many athletes and rock stars wear, since they protect your eyes from all angles. Ideally, all types of eyewear, including prescription glasses and contact lenses, should absorb the entire UV spectrum.

USING SUNSCREEN

Many people migrate to warmer climates to enjoy the outdoors. For these people, wearing clothes from head to foot to protect against intense sunlight may not be appealing, since other factors—such as heat exhaustion—may come into play. In these situations, the importance of using sunscreen cannot be stressed enough. It is especially important for children six months of age and older, who are generally the most vulnerable to UV radiation, to use sunscreen for any exposed area of skin, since UVR damage is cumulative and UV exposure at a young age greatly increases the risk of getting skin cancer later in life. Sunscreens generally should not be used for babies younger than six months since their skin is more sensitive to chemicals. Instead, small babies should be shielded from the sun and wear hats and other protective clothing.

Sunscreens come in different shapes and forms. There are sprays, lotions, creams, ointments, gels, and wax sticks. There are a number of things to consider when selecting a sunscreen. An important consideration is the **sun protection factor** (**SPF**). This represents the level of sunburn protection provided by the sunscreen from UVB, which is indicated on the label. Most sunscreens protect effectively against UVB and moderately against UVA.

It is estimated that regular application of sunscreen with a SPF of 15 or greater for the first 18 years of life reduces the lifetime incidence of nonmelanoma skin cancers by 78 percent. Sunscreens provide some protection against UV radiation but not total protection. Therefore, it is important to remember that sunscreens are not 100 percent effective and that many do not protect sufficiently against UVA.

TYPES OF SUNSCREEN

There are two types of sunscreens: physical reflectors and chemical absorbers. Physical reflectors reflect or scatter UV rays from the

TABLE 8.1 EYE PROTECTION AGAINST ULTRAVIOLET RADIATION			
TYPE OF COMMERCIALLY AVAILABLE EYEGLASSES (SUNGLASSES)	PERCENTAGE OF PROTECTION AGAINST UVA RADIATION	PERCENTAGE OF PROTECTION AGAINST UVB RADIATION	RECOMMENDED USE
Cosmetic	Gives about 20 percent eye protection	Gives about 70 percent eye protection	Good for general everyday use
General purpose	Gives about 60 percent eye protection	Gives about 95 percent eye protection	Good for out-door activities
Special purpose	Gives about 60 percent eye protection	Gives about 99 percent eye protection	Good for very bright environments

skin and are usually thick, opaque creams that are white or colored. Examples of these are zinc oxide, titanium oxide, and red petroleum. Chemical absorbers are compounds that absorb UV rays. The higher-energy short waves in UVR are absorbed by the lotion, while the remaining UV waves are converted into lower-energy long waves as they interact with the active compounds of the sunscreen. Examples are salicylates, cinnamates, Para-aminobenzoate (PABA) derivatives, and benzophenones.

It is important to read the label on the sunscreen bottle or tube to see whether the sunscreen contains physical reflectors or chemical absorbers.

Other factors to consider when buying a sunscreen include:

♦ Expiration date: The active compounds in the sunscreen degrade after a period of time (usually within two to three years). It is always important to check the expiration date on the bottle and to only use sunscreen that has not expired.

♦ Waterproof sunscreen: If you are swimming or tend to sweat a lot, a waterproof sunscreen should always be used. This will provide at least one hour of protection against UVR.

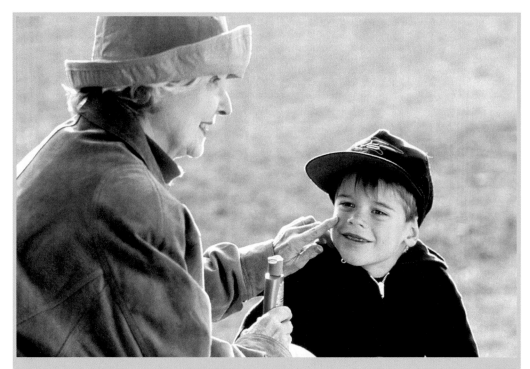

Figure 8.1   Sunscreens are important to protect us against UVR. (*National Cancer Institute/US National Institutes of Health*)

♦ Skin irritation: Sunscreens irritate some people's skin or cause them to break out in pimples, so they stop using them. There are now many products on the market that are hypoallergenic, meaning that they are designed for people with sensitive skin. The best way to find the right sunscreen for your skin is to apply a small amount on your arm for three days. If your skin does not turn red or become tender and itchy, then the sunscreen should be fine.

APPLYING SUNSCREEN

The application technique is important when putting on sunscreen. Always apply a generous helping of sunscreen to cover all sun-exposed areas. Often, people have a striped "zebra" look after coming back from vacation because they did not apply their sunscreen consistently and

TABLE 8.2   SUNSCREEN COMPOUNDS

COMPOUND GROUP	TYPE OF SUNSCREEN	PROTECTS AGAINST
PABA	Chemical absorber	UVB
Cinnamates	Chemical absorber	UVB + some UVA
Benzophenones	Chemical absorber	UVB + some UVA
Titanium dioxide	Physical reflector	UVB + UVA
Zinc oxide	Physical reflector	UVB + UVA
Salicylates	Chemical absorber	UVB
Anthranilates	Chemical absorber	UVA

◆ SUN PROTECTION FACTOR (SPF)

The SPF number system was devised to help consumers select the correct sunscreen for their skin type. The SPF number indicates the time you can normally spend in the sun without sun protection before you start to burn (this is about 20 minutes on a light-skinned person). If you multiply this number by the SPF number, this is the length of time, in minutes, that you can stay in the sun without burning. For example, SPF 15 X 20 minutes = 300 minutes in the sun without burning, which is equivalent to five hours. Therefore, the higher the SPF number, the greater the protection. SPF, however, is only a measure of the protection against UVB, not UVA. Many "broad-spectrum" sunscreens will protect against both types of UV radiation. An SPF 30 sunscreen blocks out 97 percent of the burning UV rays and is highly recommended when out in intensely bright, hot climates. There are also sunscreens with higher SPF, such as SPF 60; however, this is not thought to be that much more effective than using SPF 30. UVR exposure is also greater on reflective surfaces like water, snow, and sand, so for these high-glare situations, a higher SPF sunscreen or zinc oxide should be used on the nose and lips, which are more prominent and are therefore more exposed to UVR.

got sunburned in the areas not covered properly. It is important not only to apply sunscreen completely and evenly, but also to reapply it regularly (about every two hours), since the reaction of the sunscreen with UVR can degrade the active compounds in the sunscreen. Clothing can also rub sunscreen off the skin. More frequent applications are required when swimming. For maximum effectiveness, sunscreen should be applied 20 to 30 minutes before going outside. Also, the lips can burn and develop skin cancer so it is important to apply a sunscreen lip balm.

SUMMARY

It is relatively easy for most of us to decrease our chances of developing skin cancer. We can do this by protecting our skin from excessive sun exposure. Also, almost all skin cancers are easily detectable since the skin is a highly visible organ. A proper self-examination should be done often in front of a full-length mirror or by a doctor during a routine health examination. If something looks suspicious, it is important to visit a dermatologist, who can tell whether a mole is normal or is an early-stage skin tumor. Most life-threatening skin cancers are highly curable if detected early, so if there are any doubts about a growth, it is important to have it checked by the doctor. Remember: It is always better to prevent skin cancer than to try to cure it.

9

FUTURE PERSPECTIVES

KEY POINTS

- Understanding the underlying mechanisms of skin cancer development is important to developing new cures.

- Better education about skin cancer prevention and treatment is required to decrease the rate of skin cancer.

- Scientific and clinical research is the way forward to find newer and better ways to treat cancer.

Skin cancer is the most common cancer, and it is also the most preventable and curable form of cancer if it is detected early. The incidence of skin cancer, however, has reached epidemic proportions in the United States, with at least one million new cases of skin cancer diagnosed every year. It is estimated that one in five Americans will develop a skin cancer in his or her lifetime.

For those people who do develop skin cancer, it is reassuring to know that the majority of skin cancers (over 90 percent) can be successfully cured if discovered and treated early. As with other cancers, the longer a skin tumor is left untreated, the more likely the cancer will become more aggressive and metastasize. If metastasis occurs, the cancer is very difficult, if not impossible, to treat successfully. Therefore, for many with cancers like advanced metastatic melanoma, the outcome is poor. Patients generally die relatively quickly, sometimes in a painful way. This is certainly the case for advanced metastatic melanoma, which is a highly aggressive disease. When the metastases cause pain and discomfort for patients with advanced cancer, palliative care, radiation therapy, and pain medication are the only options to improve their quality of life.

Since there so few effective therapies that can effectively treat advanced stage cancers, more research into the biology of cancer is needed to gain a better understanding of this group of diseases. Scientists need to understand both the normal processes of tissue and organ development as well as the processes involved in cancer initiation and progression to develop better detection and treatment strategies that may improve the patient's chance of survival. Many scientists and clinicians are carrying out scientific research into the many different aspects of skin cancer. Some have focused on detection, while others have looked at chemopreventive and therapeutic drugs against skin cancer.

NEW WAYS TO TREAT SKIN CANCER

There are several new approaches to develop effective drugs against cancer. Many of these approaches target the immune system, while others try to utilize the cell machinery to trigger apoptosis. Some of the newer approaches include:

♦ Immunotherapy using leukine (GM-CSF). This molecule activates the immune system to boost the body's immune response to target tumor cells for destruction. Trials with this drug on melanoma are being carried out in the United States.

♦ Tumor vaccines. Cancer vaccines contain cell components that are only present in the tumor. These are used to "immunize" the patient, just as a flu shot will protect someone against getting the flu. This kind of therapy is being researched for several types of cancer. It may be more beneficial as a preventive therapy aimed at boosting the immune response to cancer as it begins to develop.

♦ Angiogenesis inhibitors. These agents are designed to block the growth of the new blood vessels needed to feed the growing tumor, thus cutting off the nutrient supplies so that the tumor stops growing. It is not known whether this therapy will work for metastatic cancers like melanoma. It has shown some promise in treating multiple myeloma (a cancer of the plasma cells in bone marrow), but has failed in advanced trials for lung cancer. The first angiogenesis inhibitor to be approved by the Food and Drug Administration (FDA) is Avastin (bevacizumab), for the treatment of colorectal cancer. Avastin is thought to inhibit a protein called vascular endothelial growth factor (VEGF). This protein is required for the formation of new blood vessels.

♦ Using viruses to cure skin cancer. In 2004, a group of Australian researchers reported that the Coxsackie virus—a virus that can live in the human gut and is a common cause of sore throats—can kill melanoma cells and leave normal cells intact. This is because melanoma cells have a large number of proteins on their cell surface that the virus uses to get inside cells and attack them. Human melanoma tumors grown on mice injected with Coxsackie virus disappeared within a month; however, it remains to be seen whether this type of therapy will be effective in humans.

A NEW METHOD FOR DETECTING SKIN CANCER

A report in 2004 suggested that it may be possible to carry out non-invasive detection of skin cancers by optical imaging using terahertz radiation, or T-rays. British researchers have found that T-rays, which are generated by firing a laser at a type of crystal, penetrate a few millimeters into the skin, revealing mainly surface structures, unlike X rays and MRI scans, which enter deeper into the body. T-rays are less hazardous than X rays since they do not cause as much cellular and genetic damage and can detect skin cancers such as BCCs and SCCs, which appear as darker regions on the scan. This technology could be used to assist doctors in removing tumors without taking the normal skin cells, too.

ANIMAL MODELS TO STUDY SKIN CANCER

Laboratory animals are crucial for studying diseases and finding new therapies to treat them. Much of our knowledge about the effects of UV radiation on skin comes from laboratory animal studies. Indeed, most people would object if their loved ones were being treated with therapies that have not been properly tested, and the best way to study, for example, the levels of drug toxicity, is to use an experimental animal system.

Until recently, there have been no good animal models for studying melanoma or basal cell carcinoma. As a result, our knowledge has come mainly from statistical observations of the human population and is thus incomplete. The *PATCHED1* mouse described in Chapter 4 for BCC and the *INK-4a* mouse for melanoma have proved to be valuable tools for skin cancer research. More recently, the South American opossum *Monodelphis domestica* has been suggested to be a model for the study of melanoma.

PREVENTION IS THE KEY TO CURBING MOST SKIN CANCERS

It cannot be emphasized enough that skin cancer is the most preventable cancer and that most skin cancers are caused by overexposure to UV rays in sunlight. For most people, it would not take much effort to significantly reduce the chances of developing the three main skin cancers—BCC, SCC, and melanoma. However, the notion that advanced stage melanoma and SCC may cause a rapid, painful death still does not register with "sun-worshippers," who insist that getting a glorious tan is part of what it takes to look good.

If the "sun-kissed" look is desired, there are many products on the market that will give you a tanned appearance without any UVR exposure. These fake tan products, which come as lotions or sprays, generally contain harmless dyes. When applied to the skin, they produce a deep tan that lasts several days. These products provide a safer, affordable, and convenient alternative to sunbathing and artificial tanning beds. It is important to note that even though these products give the appearance of a tan, they provide no sun protection, so people who use them should still take precautions against UVR. If the risk of dying from skin cancer still doesn't worry people, maybe having prematurely old, leathery skin that is full of wrinkles caused by excessive sun exposure may deter the image-conscious people among us!

SUMMARY

Skin cancer is the most common cancer and the most preventable. Protection against excess sun exposure is the key to prevent many of us from developing a potentially disfiguring and/or life-threatening skin cancer since there are few effective therapies for those skin cancers that have metastasized.

GLOSSARY

♦

acne   Inflammation of the sebaceous glands and hair follicles of the skin that produces pimples and pustules.

actinic keratosis   A scaly or crusty bump that forms on the skin surface. Also called solar keratosis, sun spots, or precancerous spots, since they are thought to be the earliest step in developing squamous cell carcinoma.

adjuvant therapy   Treatment given after the primary treatment to increase the chances of a cure. It may include chemotherapy, radiation therapy, hormone therapy, or biological therapy.

albinism   A rare, inherited disorder characterized by a total or partial lack of melanin (skin pigment).

anagen   The growth phase of the hair cycle during which new hair is formed.

angiogenesis   The process through which new blood vessels are formed.

antigens   Substances that cause the immune system to create antibodies.

apoptosis   Programmed cell death. Deliberate suicide of an unwanted cell in a multicellular organism.

asymptomatic   When a person does not experience symptoms.

autosomal   Relating to any one of the chromosomes except the sex chromosomes.

basement membrane   A thin, delicate layer of connective tissue underlying the epithelium of many organs.

147

benign   Not cancerous; does not invade nearby tissue or spread to other parts of the body.

biopsy   Removal of cells or tissue from a tumor for examination.

Bowen's disease   Squamous cell carcinoma *in situ*.

bulge   A location in the hair follicle that harbors the hair follicle stem cells.

calciferol   Also known as vitamin D, it is required for normal bone formation.

cancer registry   Database of cancer cases that includes information about when they occurred and the type of cancer.

carcinogen   Any substance that may cause cancer.

carcinogenesis   The process by which normal cells are transformed into cancer cells.

carcinoma   An invasive malignant tumor derived from epithelial tissue that tends to metastasize to other areas of the body.

carcinoma *in situ*   An early stage of cancer in which the tumor is confined to the site where it first develops and has not invaded other parts of the body. Most *in situ* carcinomas are highly curable.

catagen   A transitional regression phase of the hair cycle between growth and resting of the hair follicle.

chemotherapy   The use of chemical substances to treat disease.

chromosomes   Threadlike strands of DNA and associated proteins containing genetic information.

collagen   A protein that is the basic building block of connective tissues.

cyclopamine A naturally occurring chemical that is found in skunk cabbage that can cause cyclopia. It is an inhibitor of the Hedgehog signaling pathway.

deleterious Harmful or damaging.

de novo The first occurrence of cancer in the body.

desmosomes Cell structures specialized for holding cells together.

desquamation Shedding or peeling of the outer layer of the skin.

diagnosis The recognition of a disease or condition by its outward signs and symptoms.

DNA (deoxyribonucleic acid) Genetic information that contains all the information that makes us what we are.

dysplastic Abnormal cells that are not cancerous.

elastin A protein in connective tissue that is elastic and allows many tissues in the body to resume their shape after stretching or contracting.

electrodessication The drying of tissue by a high-frequency electric current applied with a needle-shaped electrode.

electromagnetic spectrum The entire range of electromagnetic radiation. The spectrum usually is divided into seven sections, from the longest wavelengths to the shortest: radio, microwave, infrared, visible, ultraviolet, X ray, and gamma ray radiation.

encapsulated Confined to a specific area.

epidemiological Referring to the study of the patterns, causes, and control of disease in groups of people.

epidermodysplasia verruciformis An autosomal recessive trait with impaired cell-mediated immunity.

epithelium   Cells that cover exterior surfaces and line internal closed cavities and exterior tube-like body structures. Epithelium also forms the secretory portion of glands and ducts.

erector pili muscles   Bundles of smooth muscle fibers, attached to the deep part of the hair follicles, passing outward alongside the sebaceous glands to the papillary layer of the dermis.

erythemal dose   The amount of radiation which, when applied to the skin, makes it turn red temporarily.

familial cancer   A cancer that runs in families.

fibroblasts   Cells that give rise to connective tissue.

free radicals   Highly reactive chemicals that often contain oxygen and are produced when molecules are split to give products that have unpaired electrons (a process called oxidation). Free radicals can damage important cellular molecules such as DNA, lipids, or other parts of the cell.

genes   Sequences of DNA that represent a fundamental unit of heredity. Most genes code for proteins.

genetic mutations   Damaged or changed regions of DNA that alter the genetic message carried by that gene.

genetic code   The set of rules by which information encoded in genetic material (DNA or RNA sequences) is translated into proteins (amino acid sequences) by living cells.

Hedgehog signaling pathway   A key regulatory pathway in animal development.

histology   The study of tissue sectioned as a thin slice.

homeostasis   The maintenance of the internal environment within tolerable limits.

horny layer   Stratum corneum. In Latin *stratum* is "layer" and *corneum* is "horny." The outer layer of the epidermis.

hyperplasia   An abnormal increase in the number of cells in a tissue or organ that is not yet a cancer.

imiquimod   A prescription medication used to treat certain diseases of the skin, including skin cancer.

immunotherapy   Treatment to stimulate or restore the ability of the immune (defense) system to fight infection and disease.

incidence   Number of newly diagnosed cases during a specific time period.

indigenous   An organism or species that both originated and evolved in a particular region.

infrared radiation   Electromagnetic radiation of wavelengths approximately between 0.75 and 1,000 nanometers, which are longer wavelengths than visible light but shorter than radio waves.

interferon   Natural proteins produced by the cells of the immune system of most vertebrates in response to challenges by foreign agents such as viruses, bacteria, parasites, and tumor cells.

interleukin-2 (IL-2)   A hormone of the immune system that is instrumental in the body's natural response to microbial infection and in discriminating between foreign and nonforeign cells.

keratin   A tough, insoluble protein substance that is the chief structural constituent of hair, nails, horns, and hooves.

keratinization   Process by which keratin is deposited in cells and the cells become "horny" (as in nails and hair).

lesions   Localized diseased or dysfunctional changes in bodily organs or tissues.

lymph   A nearly colorless fluid that bathes body cells and moves through the lymphatic vessels of the body.

lymphatic system   Network of lymph-carrying vessels and the lymphoid organs, such as the lymph nodes, spleen, and thymus, which produce and store infection-fighting cells.

lymph nodes   Bean-sized organs made up mostly of densely packed immune cells called lymphocytes, lymph fluid, and connective tissue. Clusters of lymph nodes are distributed throughout the body and are essential to a functional immune system. Lymph nodes are connected with other lymph nodes, other lymphoid tissue, and with the blood by the lymphatic vessels.

lysosomal enzymes   Enzymes that are commonly located in lysozomes that break down complex chemicals within a cell that are no longer useful.

macroscopic   Visible to the naked eye.

malignancy   Cancerous growth that may have the ability to invade, spread, and actively destroy normal tissue.

malignant   A cancerous tumor that may metastasize.

mechanoreceptors   Specialized sensory end organs that respond to mechanical stimuli such as tension, pressure, or displacement.

melanoma   A cancer of the pigment-producing cells, the melanocytes, it is the most aggressive and deadliest form of skin cancer.

mesothelioma   A malignant tumor of the mesothelium, which is the thin lining on the surface of the body cavities and the organs that are contained within them.

metaplasia   A change in cells to a form that does not normally occur in the tissue in which it is found.

metastases or **metastasis**   The spread of cancer from its primary site to other places in the body.

micrometastases   Many small metastases that are too small to be seen in a screening or test.

mitosis   The process by which a cell duplicates its genetic information (DNA) to generate two identical daughter cells with the same amount of DNA.

mitotic index   The ratio between the number of cells in mitosis and the total number of cells. It is a measure for the proliferation status of a cell population.

moles   Also known as a nevi, clusters of melanocytes that become a pigmented skin lesion.

murine   Related to mice.

mutations   Permanent changes in the DNA that can be caused by many factors, including environmental agents such as radiation and mutagenic chemicals.

neoplasm   New growth or tumor that may be benign or malignant.

neurodegenerative diseases   Diseases caused by the irreversible deterioration of essential cell and tissue components of the nervous system.

nevi   Also known as a mole, a cluster of melanocytes that becomes a pigmented skin lesion.

nonmelanoma skin cancer   Skin cancer that arises in basal cells or squamous cells but not in melanocytes.

oncogene   Genes that help cell growth and promote cancer development.

oncologist   A physician specializing in cancer diagnosis and treatment.

oncology   The study of cancer.

osteomalacia   The adult equivalent of the disease rickets.

ozone layer   The part of the earth's atmosphere that contains relatively high concentrations of ozone (O_3), which is vitally important to life because it absorbs biologically harmful ultraviolet (UV) radiation.

Pacinian corpuscles   An encapsulated receptor found in deep layers of the skin that senses vibratory pressure and touch.

palliative care   Any form of medical care or treatment that concentrates on reducing the severity of the symptoms, but is not a cure.

papillary dermis   The region closest to the epidermis that provides a strong connection between the epidermis and dermis. It contains fibroblasts that secrete collagen, elastin, and other molecules that are needed for the support and elasticity of the skin.

pathogenesis   The mechanism by which a factor causes disease.

photoaging   The process by which skin is changed or damaged as a result of exposure to ultraviolet radiation in sunlight and other sources.

plasma membrane   A thin membrane around the cytoplasm of a cell that controls the movement of substances into and out of the cell.

pluripotent   Able to develop into multiple cell types.

polymorphism   A variant form of a gene. Most polymorphisms are harmless and are part of normal human genetic variation.

preangiogenic   Before blood vessels have formed.

precursors   Biochemical substances, such as intermediate compounds in a chain of enzymatic reactions, from which more stable or definitive products are formed.

precursor lesion Localized pathological change in a bodily organ or tissue that is seen as a precancerous warning sign.

primary tumor The original tumor at the original site where it formed.

prognosis The probable outcome of a disease.

radial growth phase The early pattern of growth of cutaneous malignant melanoma in which tumor cells spread laterally (or horizontally) into the epidermis.

radiologists Physicians who specialize in radiology, the branch of medicine that uses ionizing and nonionizing radiation for the diagnosis and treatment of disease.

reticular dermis The thicker layer of the dermis that is important for the overall strength and elasticity of the skin.

rickets A disease in children resulting from a softening of the bones, potentially leading to fractures and deformity, most often as a result of vitamin D deficiency.

sarcoma A cancer that develops in connective tissues such as cartilage, bone, fat, muscle, blood vessels, and fibrous tissues (related to tendons or ligaments).

scarring A natural process in which areas of fibrous tissue replace normal skin after part of the dermis is damaged.

sebocytes Cells that produce and secrete the oily substance sebum in skin.

species A single, distinct class of living creature with features that distinguish it from others.

squamous cells Cuboidal flat cells that form the surface of an epithelium.

squamous epithelium Epithelium consisting of one or more cell layers, the most superficial of which is composed of flat, scalelike, or platelike cells.

stem cells Cells that have the ability to clone themselves and can differentiate into a wide range of specialized cell types.

stratification Formation of layers.

stratum corneum The outermost surface of the epidermis, or "horny" layer.

stratum lucidum A thin, clear layer of dead skin cells in the epidermis that is composed mainly of dead cells that lack nuclei.

sun protection factor (SPF) An indication of the time period you can stay in the sun without burning, based on your skin complexion.

symptom A sign or an indication of disorder or disease, especially when experienced by an individual as a change from normal function, sensation, or appearance.

telogen The resting phase of the hair follicle.

tonofibrils Cytoplasmic keratin protein structures in epithelial tissues that converge at desmosomes.

topical nitrogen mustard A topical chemotherapy used to treat cutaneous lymphoma.

totipotent Used to describe cells with the capacity to form an entire organism.

transiently amplifying cells Cells that divide for a limited number of times before differentiating into a mature cell type.

tumors Abnormal tissue growths that can be either benign or malignant.

tumor suppressor genes Genes that prevent cancer development.

undifferentiated   Term used to describe cells that are immature.

vaccines   Preparations of weakened or killed pathogens, such as bacteria or viruses, or of a portion of the pathogens' structure that upon administration stimulate antibody production or cellular immunity against the pathogens but are incapable of causing severe infection.

vertical growth phase   The late pattern of growth of cutaneous malignant melanoma in which tumor cells spread from the epidermis into the dermis.

wavelength   The distance between two successive points of an electromagnetic waveform (a series of electromagnetic waves), usually measured in nanometers (nm).

FURTHER RESOURCES

♦

Bibliography

Armstrong, Lance, and Sally Jenkins. *It's Not About the Bike: My Journey Back to Life.* New York: Berkley Publishing Group, 2000.

Brodland, D.G. "Diagnosis of Nonmelanoma Skin Cancer." *Clinical Dermatology* 13 (1995): 551–557.

Burston, J., and R.D. Clay. "The Problems of Histological Diagnosis in Basosquamous Cell Carcinoma of the Skin." *Journal of Clinical Pathology* 12, no. 1 (1959): 73–79.

Chambers, A.F., A.C. Groom, and I.C. MacDonald. "Dissemination and Growth of Cancer Cells in Metastatic Sites." *Nature Reviews of Cancer* 2, no. 8 (2002): 563–572.

Cooper, J.M. *The Cancer Book.* Sudbury, Mass.: Jones and Barlett Publishers, 1993.

Egan, T. *Skin Cancer: Current and Emerging Trends in Detection and Treatment.* New York: Rosen Central, 2005.

Goldberg, L.H. "Basal Cell Carcinoma." *Lancet* 347 (1996): 663–667.

Hall, H.I., K. McDavid, C.M. Jorgensen, and J.M. Craft. "Factors Associated with Sunburn in White Children Aged 6 Months to 11 Years." *American Journal of Preventive Medicine.* 20, no. 1 (January 2001): 9–14.

Halpern, A.C., and J.F. Altman. "Genetic Predisposition to Skin Cancer." *Current Opinion in Oncology* 11, no. 2 (1999): 132–138.

Kanzler, M.H., and S. Mraz-Gernhard. "Primary Cutaneous Malignant Melanoma and Its Precursor Lesions: Diagnostic and Therapeutic Overview." *Journal of the American Academy of Dermatology* 45 (2001): 260–276.

Kelvin, J. *100 Q&A About Cancer Symptoms and Cancer Treatment Side Effects.* Sudbury, Mass.: Jones and Bartlett Publishers, 2004.

Kenet, B.J, and P. Lawler. *Saving Your Skin: Prevention, Early Detection, and Treatment of Melanoma and Other Skin Cancers.* New York: Four Walls Eight Windows, 1998.

Long, W. *Coping With Melanoma and Other Skin Cancers.* New York: Rosen Publishing Group, 1999.

Marks, R. "An Overview of Skin Cancers: Incidence and Causation." *Cancer* 75, 2 suppl. (1995): 607–612.

McClay, E.F. *100 Questions and Answers About Melanoma & Other Skin Cancers.* Boston: Jones and Bartlett, 2003.

Ratner, Désirée, M.D. "Commentary: New Developments in Cutaneous Oncology" *Clinics in Dermatology.* 22, no. 3 (May-June 2004): 175–177.

Rodden, Robinson, T. *Genetics for Dummies.* Hoboken, N.J.: John Wiley & Sons, Inc., 2005.

Shaath, N.A. *Sunscreens: Regulation and Commercial Development*, 3d ed. White Plains, N.Y.: Marcel Dekker, 2005.

Schalick, W.O. "History of basal cell carcinoma." In: *Cutaneous Oncology: Pathophysiology, Diagnosis, and Management.* Miller S. J. and Maloney M.E., eds. Malden, Mass.: Blackwell Science, 1998: 578–80.

Web Sites

American Academy of Dermatology
http://www.aad.org/

American Cancer Society
http://www.cancer.org/

American Joint Committee on Cancer: Cancer Staging
http://www.cancerstaging.org/

Association of International Cancer Research (United Kingdom-based charity organization)
http://www.aicr.org.uk/index.stm

Basal Cell Nevus Syndrome Support Group (USA)
http://www.bccns.org/nbccs.htm

The Cancer Council Australia (official Australian cancer and cancer prevention organization)
http://www.cancer.org.au/

Center of Disease Control and Prevention (CDC) US Department of Health and Human Services skin cancer information
http://www.cdc.gov/cancer/skin/pdf/sknaag01.pdf

Clinical Trials for Cancer
http://www.clinicaltrials.gov/

Environmental Protection Agency
http://www.epa.gov/sunwise/uvandhealth.html

Food and Drug Administration (FDA)
http://www.fda.gov

Federal Trade Commission: Tanning Information
http://www.ftc.gov/bcp/edu/pubs/consumer/health/heal1.shtm

Howard Hughes Medical Institute (discovery of the mutation that causes BCNS)
http://www.hhmi.org/genesweshare/b220.html

International Union Against Cancer (UICC)
http://www.uicc.org/

National Cancer Institute (NCI)
http://www.cancer.gov/

National Center for Biotechnology Information
http://www.ncbi.nlm.nih.gov

National Institute of Allergies and Infectious Diseases, National Institute of Health (Human Papillomavirus and Genital Warts)
http://www.niaid.nih.gov/factsheets/stdhpv.htm

National Institutes of Health
http://www.nih.gov/

Online Emergency Medicine magazine
http://www.emedmag.com/html/pre/cov/covers/071502.asp

The Skin Cancer Foundation
http://www.skincancer.org/

"The Girl Who Lives In The Dark" (Documentary about a person with XP)
http://www.enhancetv.com.au/shop/product.php?productid=103822

The Sun Safety Alliance (SSA) (sun protection information)
http://www.sunsafetyalliance.org/

Surveillance, Epidemiology and End Results (SEER) program—the official source of statistical information used by the National Cancer Institute (NCI)
http://seer.cancer.gov/data/

Cancer Staging
http://www.cancer.gov/cancertopics/factsheet/Detection/tumor-grade

General skin cancer information at University of California San Francisco (UCSF)
http://dermatology.ucsf.edu/preview/skincancer/

World Health Organization
www.who.int

INDEX

♦

ABOUT THE AUTHOR

◆

PO-LIN SO received her bachelor's degree in genetics from Queen Mary College, University of London, and a Ph.D. in developmental biology from King's College, University of London. Her studies focused on the biological and therapeutic roles of vitamin A derivatives in the developing embryo and in the adult nervous system. More recently, as an assistant researcher at the University of California, San Francisco, she has focused on understanding the biological complexities of skin cancer—more specifically, how genes that are important in the development of the embryo and the nervous system play a role in cancer development. Her research also focuses on the identification of potential preventive and therapeutic therapies to treat skin cancer. She is currently continuing her research as an assistant staff scientist at Children's Hospital Oakland Research Institute.